FAT

The Body, Food *and* Obesity

DR ISHRAT SYED

DR KALPANA SWAMINATHAN

SPEAKING TIGER

SPEAKING TIGER PUBLISHING PVT. LTD
4381/4, Ansari Road, Daryaganj
New Delhi 110002

First published in paperback by Speaking Tiger 2018

ISBN: 978-93-88326-20-9
eISBN: 978-93-88326-21-6

10 9 8 7 6 5 4 3 2 1

Typeset in Sabon Roman by SÜRYA, New Delhi
Printed at Nutech Print Services - India

Dr Ishrat Syed is a general and paediatric surgeon. As photographer he uses the camera to explore hidden histories.

Dr Kalpana Swaminathan is a paediatric surgeon. She won the 2009 Crossword Award for *Venus Crossing: Twelve Stories of Transit*.

They write together as Kalpish Ratna. Their last book was *The Secret Life of Zika Virus* (2017).

for

Shakir Ali Syed

2 July 1928, Nagina – 16 August 2017, Bombay

In Memoriam

CONTENTS

Part 1

MECHANISMS

The Body Blog

If I were to ask, 'What does your body look like?' your answer will describe how you see yourself. This may, or may not, match what the mirror shows.

If I asked, 'What does your body feel like?' you would probably pause.

Your reply might be polite and noncommittal.

Or, it might be a literal descriptor of aches, pains, discomforts, if you're feeling unwell.

In either case, your reply is scarcely as revealing as the pause that preceded it. In that pause, you *noticed* your body in a manner unusual for you.

What was so unusual about that perception?

The usual modus vivendi with which we perceive our bodies is visual.

We think, practically all the time, about what we look like.

The self self-image either matches or fails to match the ideal we would like to project. And that ideal—however vociferously we may deny it—is shaped by circumstance.

Circumstances of birth, culture, society, peer pressure, all collude to create a mould that is the archetype for success/happiness/acceptance.

Your perception of your body may either conform to this mould or shatter it with a vengeance. Either way, it is shaped by factors external to you.

Factors internal to you only become noticeable when you're ill.

A stomach ache tells you there's something happening in the hidden compartment beneath your belt.

A headache can make you frighteningly aware of your brain.

And what conspiracy of demons is making your back a living hell?

All illness carries a heavy burden of dread. That's because discomfort startles you into defying a taboo.

You are forced to acknowledge that the body is NOT skin deep.

The skin, our marvellous gift wrapping, is so attractive, so sentient, so efficient, and taken so much for granted, that a breach in its seamless continuity can be simply terrifying. Even a small wound, the merest laceration, can disturb us, way beyond the immediate distress of pain and bleeding.

We're disturbed by that sudden peek into the gaping lips of a wound.

We prefer not to think of what lies beneath, and so we hastily look away.

It isn't as if our insides aren't making themselves heard. They issue status reports at regular intervals, but we acknowledge none of them until they're past ignoring—and *then* they are embarrassments.

We cough, sneeze, burp, fart, rumble.

We ache, tingle, cramp up.

We flush with unexpected thrills of desire.

How many of these signals are *polite*?

How many of these do we hastily suppress in public?

Remember that old chestnut? That man is a social animal, and woman even more so?

The steep slope from savage to civilized involves an erasure of the body at each step.

It is interesting to examine how magical these erasures are. We can track them through religion and ritual, through superstition, shibboleth and lore.

The body continues to embarrass. Like a Victorian child, it may be seen but not heard.

This taboo seems destined to remain. The body must not be fitted into the mind's domain.

But it already is! The brain is hardwired into understanding every cell of your body—trillions of them. It is reading their tweets constantly.

Why not then break this taboo right now?

Stop at this sentence and give yourself a beat of silence.

Your body's signals will twinkle, glimmer, and soon glare into view.

That tight feeling on your shoulders demands a shift to a more comfortable seat perhaps? A cushion?

That tingling in your toes tells you your legs need to swing free. Might as well investigate the fridge if you're going to get up, find a bite of something tasty, and hey, how about some music while you quick-step to the bathroom and back?

See what I mean?

That little break refreshed you. And no, it wasn't 'just psychological'.

'Feel good' is not about the ersatz high you get from an hour at the gym, or prayer, or gossip, or whatever. It is about taking charge of your life by accepting responsibility for your body.

Your body is the only piece of real estate you'll ever indisputably own. It dies with you. Whatever your belief may be, there is no factual proof that there is an afterlife.

This is all you have, this moment, this lifetime in an incredibly sophisticated, beautiful home with mod cons beyond the wildest of dreams. And it is absolutely rent free. Why not wallow in this climate-controlled luxury suite while you enjoy the view?

All it requires is a conversation between your body and you.

The Big O

Obesity is trending now, and nobody, it seems, wants to be left behind.

Out on the street, obesity stares us in the face. It is a *visual* label.

The O word is seldom uttered. Most people would consider it body shaming.

It can be nuanced: *I'm healthy, you're plump, he's overweight, she's fat, they're obese.*

Inevitable, in today's lookist society. Even more so in a nation with a recent memory of want.

To most Indians, body weight is a measure of worth.

Today's plutocrat might think twice about tulabharam, the ancient royal custom where the ruler was weighed in gold and silver and the coin distributed in charity. On a more plebeian scale, embonpoint is a covetable social asset. It separates the arriviste, the gate crasher, the mleccha from the blue-blooded scions of a *khata-peeta khandan*.

This belief is probably a fall-out of the nineteenth century when you had to be a really well-heeled hoarder to stay fat through famine after famine under Victoria's benign reign. Seventy years of independence and we are still a hairsbreadth away from starvation.

In ancient India, fat was never fashionable. That truth is cut in stone. The human body is celebrated in sculpture everywhere on the subcontinent. The forms may be idealized—but not without the occasional nod to realism.

In Kanheri Caves, the sculptor has left a sardonic comment. Next to gracile apsaras and bodhisattvas, there is a a very earthy tableau. He has sculpted a fleshy, paunchy group of men and women who clearly grossed him out. Rich donors, probably, who left his bill unpaid. And that lampoon is from the sixth century.

Further back in time are the hoary Samhitas of Charaka and Sushruta which form the core of Ayurveda. In these medical texts, obesity is called atisthulyam. It is described and diagnosed as a disease.

Atisthulyam is regarded as dangerous, its complications as potentially fatal.

The ancient understanding of the disorders of obesity is startlingly modern. It is defined as a disorder of metabolism in which fat tissue (meda) increases at the cost of depriving other essential tissues (dhatu) of energy. This was the Indian outlook on obesity in 1500 B.C.

Yet, till 2013, Indians, like the rest of the world, insisted on viewing obesity as a purely cosmetic problem.

Fat is something that makes you look bad, so get it fixed!

To our eternal shame, qualified doctors, especially surgeons, embraced this diktat by mindlessly and obsessively scooping out wads of fat through lipectomies, liposuction, and like procedures.

The marketing cool played perfectly into narcissism. The sell was for 'body-sculpting'. The O word was carefully edited out.

Could the fitness industry be far behind? Diets, exercises, wraps, vapour baths, massages, an alternative pharmacy from every world culture—we ran through them all, panting, for several decades.

And, we simply got fatter.

Every doctor worth her or his salt since Sushruta knows the hazards an obese patient faces. It was not until four years ago, in 2013, that obesity's metabolic profile received official recognition.

So finally, we can dump the guilt, and get honest about obesity.

It is not about how we *look*.

It is about we *feel*.

Tired. Irritable. Out of breath. Creaking at every joint. Hungry, and miserable about being hungry.

It can't all be 'psychological'.

Something must be radically wrong.

And it is.

Obesity is a low energy state.

'Metabolism' is what keeps the body alive—the process of changing the food we eat into the energy needed by each of the body's myriad cells. This is disordered in most overweight people. This changed metabolism causes complications ranging from trivial discomforts to frequent illnesses, to established diseases that can maim or kill. Because these complications are multifarious, they are conveniently bracketed as a syndrome. Being overweight finally gets a scientific label: *Metabolic Syndrome*.

In 1500 B.C. Sushruta pointed out what we see every day. The abdomen is a fat depot. In obesity, abdominal fat increases dramatically.

Put plainly, one has a paunch.

And, the wobble in the t-shirt is an iceberg—7/8th packed out of sight inside the abdominal cavity.

Today, the official description of Metabolic Syndrome specifies abdominal obesity and links it with another fact Sushruta made a big deal about: *dyslipidemia*, or the alteration in blood fats.

A third factor that is very significant to us today is high blood pressure.

17.7 million people die of cardiovascular diseases every

year. Most of them have Metabolic Syndrome. The tag in itself means nothing, but it explains what happens within the body when we're feeling fat.

How can a condition so common be so frightening?

How did so frightening a condition become so common?

Why now? We have been eating like this for centuries, so how come, all of a sudden, we're a fat nation now?

Yes, we are.

It isn't just the coffee shop and the pizzeria crowd. We are also talking aam aadmi and aurat, the gharelu feeders, the daal-roti, thayir-chadam crowd. Metromental? Not at all, we are rural too. Fat Nation, WE.

And so what?

Can't one be both fat *and* fit?

Thousands of us apparently are. We go about a strenuous and hectic life with extra kilos strapped on us, just as children do with their heavy school bags, and seem none the worse for it.

'Seem' is the operative word.

Neither the child who labours under a heavy bag, nor an adult who strains under the burden of extra weight, escapes bodily damage.

Our understanding of this has been very slow, and is still very far from perfect. Even the recognition of Metabolic Syndrome as a disease process has been painfully reluctant, discrediting the *experience* of feeling fat.

What changes in us to make us feel different when we're fat?

Here is a simple analogy.

The body is demonetized. Every cell in the body needs energy to function. The body's currency is a molecule called Adenosine Triphosphate, ATP. It is produced from the food we eat through a cascade of biochemical reactions.

When we get fat, the conversion of food to energy is

blocked, and the cell is starved of immediate currency. Instead, the food is converted into more fat.

When this happens, the body then breaks down its own tissues to provide energy for cell processes. This results in an actual *loss* of lean body mass—muscle, bone, blood, and body organs are all in a state of constant breakdown to provide the energy needed for us to keep ticking. Meanwhile, we keep eating, and keep piling on fat.

As we recently learnt in the political arena, in the aftermath of demonetization, the economy eventually caves in.

Factually, the cardiovascular system is the commonest target. The 'fit fat' group are more prone to heart attacks and strokes than the normal weight population. The heart and its groupies aren't the only victims—bones and joints, the liver and the blood, also sign in sick.

Why does this happen?

Why should the impact of obesity be so widespread in the body?

The term Metabolic Syndrome gathers all these various miseries under its umbrella in an attempt to discover a common denominator.

Structurally, that denominator is fat.

So what is fat?

Is the fat in the body the same stuff we use to fry puri?

Yes and no.

Fat, biochemically, is an ester of fatty acid and glycerol. All fat, anywhere—animal, vegetable or mineral—has this composition.

Body fat, also called adipose tissue, is a little more complex than cooking oil because it is present within living cells and is therefore constantly dynamic.

Fat is not quite the placid couch potato it is made out to be. It is in hectic overdrive.

What is happening in that soft and delicate luxurious lining just beneath the skin?

Dermis Deluxe

'Ain't he fit to bust out of his clothes, and start the seams, and make the very buttons fly off with his fatness? Here's flesh!' cried Squeers, turning the boy about, and indenting the plumpest parts of his figure with divers pokes and punches, to the great discomposure of his son and heir. 'Here's firmness, here's solidness! Why you can hardly get up enough of him between your finger and thumb to pinch him anywheres.'

—Charles Dickens,
The Life and Adventures of Nicholas Nickleby

Close your eyes and think luxury couture.

What do you see? Silks and velvets? Fur and feathers?

Me, I prefer something more sensuous. Soft, supple, moulded to contours round or angled, rippling subtly with movement, yet tenacious in embrace. A fabric so sentient it translates the world for me. It is impeccably bespoke. Nobody else will ever wear it. It is as plebeian as pret will ever get. I wake up in it, sweat my six-mile walk in it, breeze out confidently to work in it. As leisure wear and pleasure wear, nonpareil. Totally undemanding too. Hand wash, towel dry. I could live in it all my life.

And, I do.

Nothing is as luxurious as skin.

That touch of luxury has nothing to do with the cosmetic expanse on view. The voluptuous glide of skin depends entirely on its invisible lining. Fatty tissue.

Fat.

The word is rooted in luxury.

Its origins, Germanic, Sanskrit, or Greek as you please, suggest a wealth of excess. *Peie, payate, poid*—to abound in water, milk, fat, etc.

The soft, resilient dimple a fingertip makes on skin is merely pleasant. The tissue that permits this pleasure is spectacular. Fat is one of the body's more amazing tissues, and probably the most misunderstood. It is dyed deep in villainy these days. Before we judge, why not get to know it?

Lest you imagine fat to be a kind of sandwich spread between skin and muscle and bone, let me quickly tell you it is a miracle of packaging. Running the fingertip along a layer of fatty tissue leaves no more than the faintest slick. Hard to believe you've been handling oil.

That's exactly what fatty tissue is. *Oil.*

The chemical content of body fat is triacylglycerol, or more snappily, TAG. As the name suggests, it's composed of three fatty acids linked to one molecule of glycerol. TAG is a *triglyceride.*

The more genteel name for body fat is *adipose tissue.* Its Latin origins are much ruder. *Adiposus* is lard.

And *tissue* derives from *texere,* to *weave.*

That is a truly literal descriptor. Body fat is a *textile* created from oil. It is sustainable luxury at its premium.

In the fashion industry, sustainable luxury is the current oxymoron. It is art calculated to engage and disturb by opening a new dimension of experience. Its motif is increasingly eco-friendly. The ethic of sustainable luxury in couture addresses the twinned misery destroying the planet: the exploitation of human beings and destruction of the environment. Hence the credo, however sincere, of no sweat shops and no cruelty to animals. Hence recycling, the motive force of a circular economy that puts back what it takes.

Believe you me, the human body works this principle into its luxury textile. Fat is all about circular economy.

Fat tissue is power dressing, but not in the way we think. Having a lot of fat, or having too little, impoverishes the body equally. Think velvet: too shaggy a pile transforms it from couture to carpet. Too sparse, and it just won't drape elegantly. But with just the right depth of give, both velvet and skin make a statement of worth and probity. To echo Mr Squeers, 'Here's richness! Here's luxury!'

And yet, body fat is oil, the same stuff that lights a lamp, fuels a car, fries a samosa and kills marine life.

Fluid and unctuous, its insidious ooze is treacherously slippery, offensively sticky, notoriously messy, and, even after a vigorous scrub, persistent as memory. Dirt finds it so irresistibly magnetic, and it stains so deep and quick, and the human loathing of these qualities is so visceral, that it sustains the 200-billion-dollar laundry detergent industry.

How does something that seems so intrinsically nasty become a textile of unsurpassable beauty, so seductive to the touch, so sublime in its drape? And, (though this is going to take some convincing) practically as intelligent as the brain?

The trick is in the packaging. Adipose tissue has all that oil packed neatly inside very special cells called *adipocytes*. The way we shudder at fat makes it seem like garbage the body can't junk fast enough. That is grave injustice to the billions of adipocytes we carry around so elegantly.

The adipocyte is an energetic, curious, reactive cell that's on the job 24/7. The image of adipose tissue as an inert slab of fat is just bad press. The fat it contains is far from inert.

Body fat is a very high energy source. It is survival food.

Each gramme of body fat yields 9 calories of energy.

An adult man of average weight has about 12 kg of adipose tissue. That is energy enough to tide him over a week of starvation.

Great—if we were starving. But when we aren't, why do we need this hoard? It seems miserly to lock up so much energy.

It isn't quite locked up.

The adipocyte keeps this energy reserve dynamic. It's constantly being broken down and replaced to meet the body's changing demands and our changing food intake.

The adipocyte is the barometer of the body's internal milieu.

You wouldn't think a nubbin of fat on the inside of your forearm would care at all about that second scoop of chocolate ice-cream.

But it does.

It has broadcast the news to the rest of the body before the ice-cream has even melted. Every organ is interested in this kind of low gossip. Bigwigs like the liver and pancreas depend on these bulletins from adipose tissue to function normally. So do your muscles. And the process of digesting that ice-cream is closely watched by the adipocyte.

Incredible?

It isn't stretching it to say adipose tissue even controls the mind.

It may not be as pretty as skin, but fat has undeniable *je ne sais quoi*. Its exuberant yellow grosses out the fastidious, and not everybody cares for its bouclé texture. Its wet-look sheen is distinctly retro. Nonetheless, it has moxie.

So it's a bit disappointing when you plan a more respectful scrutiny. A section of adipose tissue under the microscope looks—empty. It has the desolation of an abandoned city. Rows and rows of houses with walls enclosing nothing at all. No, look, there's furniture pushed against the walls, making a dark nidus inside every empty cell.

'Signet cell appearance' a medical student might confidently call it.

It is an illusion.

The usually employed stain* doesn't colour fat. A special dye like Sudan III shows up something very different. Gone is the bubble-wrap vacuity. Adiposity bulges into view as gigantic drops of oil.

This is the commonest kind of fatty tissue. Every cell is filled by a single massive drop of fat. It has a snappy name too: WAT, acronym for *White Adipose Tissue*. It isn't particularly white, but it suggests there's another darker sort as well. Predictably, that's called BAT, *Brown Adipose Tissue*. If this is not enough, there are recruit adipocytes which are called 'brite' or 'beige'. These are WATs that can transition into BATs.

And that's just the adipose tissue beneath the skin that we've been admiring. It makes up the body's reserve of *Subcutaneous Adipose Tissue*, SAT for short. There is another fat depot we carry around besides this one. It's stationed within the body cavities, cushioning the organs and great vessels. These adipocytes are in a different league altogether. They make up *Visceral Adipose Tissue*. You guessed it—VAT.

This book is an exploration of the tormented love affair between food on the plate and fat in the body. Like all great love stories, this one too is a tragedy.

> *Two households, both alike in in dignity,*
> ...
> *From ancient grudge break to new mutiny,*

A familiar trope, and a new twist of anguish, that turns romance into tragedy. And, before we examine *the fearful passage of their death-mark'd love*, let us meet the people in the play.

---

*Hematoxylin and Eosin (H&E) stain. Hematoxylin is a dye that is derived from the bloodwood tree, *Haematoxylum campechianum* (Greek *haima* = blood and *xylon* = wood). Eosin derives from the ancient Greek goddess of the dawn, Eos. Eosins are fluorescent acidic compounds that combine with proteins to stain them red or pink.

Masquerade

In a play, 'Dramatis Personæ' introduces characters by name and provenance. The body's tale is more masquerade than play. Here then are the masked players, strutting their stuff. As this book unfolds, plot and counterplot, trysts and betrayals will make these characters drop their masks, and race towards the tragic denouement, the misshapen chaos of well-seeming forms... Obesity.

The Mouth

This charming braggart is more than a bite-chew-swallow muscle machine. It can turn, within seconds, from savage to subtle, from mindless glutton to sophisticated gourmet.

With the mouth you never know. Watch it go from dental to mental.

The Food Pipe (Oesophagus)*

Is just that, a simple tube that carries what you swallow down to your stomach. It lurks at the back of your chest, silent and unnoticed, until a moment's indiscretion stabs you with heartburn.

The Stomach

This neat tote in the left side of the abdomen, tucked beneath your ribs and midriff, is brilliantly adventurous, and

*From the Greek, *oisein*, future infinitive of *pherein*, to carry, + *-phagos*, from *phagein*, to eat.

generously expansile. You can pack in all you want without fear of it bursting. Invisible and non-intrusive in its career as food processor, its acid comments on your lifestyle can hurt like hell.

The Small Intestine

Seems just a waste of space. Twenty feet of tubing to manage your modest meal? It is twitchy all the time, it spins the digested food like a jacuzzi and towels it with its absorptive deep-pile lining.

A great Turkish bath, and yes, the good stuff has all been neatly transferred into your circulation. But, there's more to its story...

The Large Intestine

This in-built sewer has always been one of the body's unmentionables, but guess what, recent research gives more status to flatus.

Everything that happens within this 5-foot trombone is a health broadcast, so watch out when it is out of tune.

The gut *microbiome* is encamped here. This is an intelligence network that answers directly to the brain.

The Liver and Gall Bladder

The liver is a thing apart from the digestive tract, but digestion would be impossible without it. Massive and kingly, it is enthroned beneath the ribs on the right side, and is practically invisible. Its secretive functions keep us alive.

Overtly, it produces bile, and stores it in an elegant pear-shaped handbag, the gall bladder.

Bile is a yellow alkaline liquid that is vital to the digestion and absorption of fat, and the gall bladder conveys it into the small intestine.

But bile does more than help break down the butter on your toast—it controls that popular demon—cholesterol.

Despite its massive arrogance, the liver is terribly sensitive. It is quickly upset as the love affair sours...

The Pancreas

The mystery organ, unseen, unfelt, its public image is DIABETES. That's the most unkindest cut of all when its principal messenger, the hormone Insulin, plays Cupid in this romance.

Insulin

This adorable molecule feeds every cell in the body by making it possible for glucose from our food to be utilized as energy. It keeps us nimble and fit. So, when the door is slammed on Insulin, the cell starves, and our little Cupid goes into a sulk.

The Muscles

These tough guys actually smooth corners and do much of the tactful family negotiations between food and fat, to the extent of sacrificing themselves when things begin to sour.

The Immune System

The body's House-keeping Department. It works 24/7. But the staff gets rebellious, and sometimes stoops to base treachery.

The Heart and Blood Vessels

The throb and pulse of life sings joyous as springtime. But misunderstandings build up sneakily, narrow the outlook, and raise suspicion...

It simmers, it simmers.

And then—heartbreak.

The Brain

The Brain keeps itself exclusive. Its ivory tower is a delicate tissue formed of special cells that wall off the blood in the capillaries. This is the Blood-Brain-Barrier (B-B-B). If the brain is so isolated, how does it run the show?

There are trysting places, where the B-B-B is either absent or simply looks the other way.

At these places, there is a rapid exchange of news between the brain and the rest of the body.

The brain is the playwright of this romance, but it is in two minds about the script.

One part of the brain ensures we *eat* to live.

The other makes us *live* to eat.

The first is the daal-chawal, roti-sabzi unit. It is all about appetite and satiety. It is about *how much*.

The other part of the brain is equally about fine dining and pigging out. It veers between pleasure and greed. It is about cravings, impulses and passions. What does it want? It answers that question with two words: sugar and fat.

Which way will the script turn?*

Hormones†

Hormones make up the live band which orchestrates life, and the Food-Fat story has some great music. The Brain conducts this symphony.

Hormones are messenger chemicals secreted directly into the bloodstream. They regulate metabolism. There are too many of them to be listed here, but they'll show up as you read on.

---

*Peters, A., & Langemann, D. (2009): 'Build-Ups in the Supply Chain of the Brain: On the Neuroenergetic Cause of Obesity and Type 2 Diabetes Mellitus.' *Frontiers in Neuroenergetics*, 1, 2. http://doi.org/10.3389/neuro.14.002.2009.

†From the Greek *hormē*, impulse, to set in motion, to urge on.

How to Grow a Brain

We are the fattest species on earth. To become human, we grew a brain, shrank the intestine, and cushioned ourselves in adipose tissue.

The evolution of the brain is obvious: intelligence explains our swagger. The intestine shrank as our ancestors ate their way through a changing landscape.

But why pile on fat?

As an evolutionary decision, it seems out of sync with the emergent species. *Homo erectus,* 1.8 mya (million years ago), was an aggressive arriviste. Smart, and with a recently increased hat size. Mobile, with enough swing in his stride to consider making it out of Africa. Wired with the latest gizmos. The newest hunter-gatherer kit was really neat, you could brain an antelope *and* skin it with the same tool. Cultured? Well, almost. There is also some evidence—only some—that *H. erectus* cooked on weekends.

Why pick boudoir chic as power dressing?

In our thanatophilic times, the story of human evolution restores sanity. It reminds us life is a hard-won right. Its narrative is the body, during life, and after death. It trades on evidence, not belief, and this evidence is tangible. Its interpretations are pluralistic, its memory is retrievable. Above all, it reconnects us with the present moment.

Our belief in the afterlife has distanced us from the reality of life. It has championed human destructiveness and caused species insurrection that imperils our survival. Not only by our compulsion to injure and kill our fellow humans, but by our pillage and plunder of the planet. We have changed the seasons with the violence of our hate.

To recover, we need to forswear disguises, we need to repudiate caste, colour and religion.

We are a species, and we must return to our identity as *Homo sapiens sapiens,* and evolve, with a little more intelligence and much less greed, towards enlightenment by cherishing the earth that sustains us.

The narrative that won us species status is located in our body, and it is all about fat.

The narrative that will destroy us is also located in our body, and it, also, is mostly about fat.

The Big O has a memory at least two million years old.

Fat makes up 15–20 per cent of body weight in us modern humans. Other terrestrial mammals have considerably less, and most don't even make it to two figures.

Yes, we have competition: hibernating bears and whales.

Still, we're fatter than our ancestors, and fatter than our nearest evolutionary cousins, the great apes.

We are born fat. Human babies are cuter than puppies and kittens because they are much fatter, and with very good reason.

A baby's brain is about 380 gm at birth. It triples in the first year, and continues to increase through early childhood. Which is to say, brain development is not complete at birth, but is completed through infancy and early childhood.

The infant brain uses up nearly 75 per cent of the body's daily energy expenditure.

In an adult, this slows down, but, considering its size (a mere 1.3 kg in an adult male of 60 kg), the brain is still a big eater. It uses up 23 per cent of the day's energy.

Thought is a hectic process. It involves a bizarre number of neurons, each one of which has to expend quite a bit of energy in the process of excitation and transmission to achieve cognition, the catch-all term for the entire gamut that makes us human—conscious thought, reason and perception.

The brain takes a lot of sugar in its coffee—up to 100 gm of glucose every day.

What if starvation strikes?

We know, from human experience, that the brain does not shut down.

From where does the brain get its energy?

It does not have a ready store of sugar. At best, the liver can mobilize its stores*—but that would last no more than a day. How does the starving body whistle up enough energy to keep the ravenous brain functioning?

From fat.

When fatty acids reach the liver, they are converted into ketones. These high energy compounds make up the brain's back-up fuel. In the foetus and infant, ketones are also building blocks for the lipids in developing brain tissue.

Fat, at various structural levels, makes up 60 per cent of the brain.

It takes a great deal of fat to build a brain and a terrific amount of energy to run it.

So, as hominins began the journey towards sapience, food had to be organized for a two-million-year-long journey. During this time, the brain would increase from 600 gm to the present 1.35 kg as we upcycled an ape-ish intelligence into the refinements of reason, language and art.

How did our ancestors manage a steady supply of nutrients for such exuberant brain growth?

Evolution had chugged along towards *Homo sapiens* for several million years, why did things accelerate, abruptly, two million years ago? When the entire planet was an extended buffet of leaves and fruit, why abandon a laid-back arboreal existence to take potshots at fleeing meat?

---

*Sugar is stored as glycogen in the liver.

Climate change.

Africa, the motherland of our species, changed from lush rainforest to woodland and savannah (Plio-Pleistocene boundary, 1.8–2 mya. There were fewer trees, and more grazers. Naturally, the menu widened. *Homo habilis*, 2 mya, has left us a tool kit as evidence.

A lot of hard work came before he could use that kit.

Lunch had a disconcerting habit of whizzing past at several miles per hour, and it had to be pursued. Long treks meant infrequent meals, but *Homo* had acquired a taste for small but rich meals. Specifically, they were rich in the nutrients required for building a larger brain.

By 1.6 mya, there is evidence of central kitchens and communal meals. The tool kit is more sophisticated now. The brain has grown by 300 gm.

Two fats are most essential to brain development. Both are long-chain polyunsaturated fatty acids. They have jawbreaker names—Docosahexaenoic acid (DHA) and Arachidonic Acid (AA). These molecules cannot be synthesized by the body. *They have to be eaten.*

From *Homo habilis* to *Homo erectus*, the brain had grown by 300 gm. This required a rich content of DHA and AA in the menu.

Fruit and leaves and tubers provide only a trace of these magic molecules, so they must have been sourced from prey.

The richest dietary source for DHA and AA is aquatic life.

Did we depend mainly on fish and other sea food to grow the brain we have today? Was evolution a coastal phenomenon?

Not only did we increase in brain size, we increased in body weight too—preferentially in fat.

Fat deposition begins before birth. From the third trimester on, the foetus begins to accumulate fat to power brain development. This continues through infancy and early childhood. These fat stores are not depleted even during starvation. The malnourished toddler is stunted in growth, but retains her fat to provide fuel for the brain.

It is not difficult to understand how this logic brought about an increase in body fat through evolution. It was to ensure that the brain had back-up fuel during food scarcity.

When lean times set in, fat is mobilized from adipose tissue as fatty acids. The liver processes these into ketones, which the brain utilizes as fuel. Without enough adipose tissue reserve, this wouldn't be possible.

Think of that incredible stretch of time—two million years—and the even more incredible complexity of the brain that we grew during this time. Now think of the incalculable energy it has cost us!

Reason enough for *Homo habilis* to have decided to grow fat *before* getting smarter.

And reason enough for us to respect our adipose tissue.

This accord endured unchallenged for two megennia. Then, in the last two hundred years, we turned it into discord.

The Changing Paradigm

Most of our information about ourselves comes to us via Western literature. It took an American study to alert us to the self-evident fact that we have a different body structure from Europeans.

Yes, when good Indians die they do go to California, but once there we do not change enough to mimic the Caucasian response to a high-fat high-protein Westernized diet. Even if we continue our shudha shakahari ways, we are bedazzled by the availability of convenience foods: sugar-loaded cereals and juices, fat-loaded bakery products, everything creamy and glistening with corn syrup.

Ouch!

Asian-Americans fall prey to cardiovascular disease and diabetes quicker than their European compatriots.

Ever since the United States recognized the dangers of trans fats and corn syrup, Indian supermarket shelves began to groan under the weight of their surplus.

Yesterday I was held up at the checkout counter in the supermarket by a couple shopping for ghar ka khana.

They were young, they would confess to forty in a year or two. A double-income nuclear family, with two kids between five and ten, judging from the shopping that was taking more than half an hour to bill.

The mountain of tinsel in their trolley took forever to dislodge, there was always one packet more to add to the pile. Everything crisp and crunchy was represented. Many of the packets, I noticed, carried the triumphant label 'baked, not fried'. There was a small hillock of high-fibre stuff for the parents, the many sorts of bhoosa-biscuit that are all the rage.

Three large consignments of cheese: blocks, wedges, slices, in addition to jars of spread.

Several gigantic bottles of fizzy drinks.

Presumably this was not the rice, atta, vegetable jaunt, but they had made minuscule purchases of daal.

A five-litre can of 'heart-healthy' cooking oil, a kilo of butter, and one of ghee hid behind a wall of many kinds of pasta.

They had one more trolley, full of toiletries.

Husband and wife peered anxiously around, scanning the shelves to see what they had forgotten.

From their conversation it was obvious they were loving and concerned parents, responsible householders, pleasant people—

And yet, they were going home with *this*.

With Diwali round the corner, the market is rabid with clothing sales. Looking for a gift for my petite niece, I join the buzz around a kurti display. The designs are imaginative, the colours delightful, but the sizes—

This year's styles have flowing lines, delicate pastels almost vaporous in drift on the mannequins outside. But when the salesman holds up the kurti I've picked, it seems as large as a tent.

Suddenly everybody else wants it too.

The din is indescribable.

The salesman, helpless against the barrage, pulls down a fresh lot of merchandise.

A plaintive voice cuts through the clamour. My heart sinks as I realize it is my own. 'Don't you have a smaller size?'

In the beat of silence that follows, two things happen.

The woman at my elbow gives a short scornful laugh.

The salesman chooses to answer my question. 'Chalta nahi. Only XL and XXL.'

Eventually, I'm trotted around to a small, sorry selection so outdated, it is almost historic.

'These are out of fashion,' I point out.

The salesman shrugs. 'Only XL and XXL are in fashion. That's what public wants.'

'Only some,' I protest.

'No, no. It is normal. XL is normal. XXL maybe not so much, maybe fifty percent.'

Like the emperor's famous new clothes, obesity is invisible. The danger with this genre of invisibility is that it quickly establishes a new norm.

The scariest word I know is *normal*. Who sets the norm?

I faced this question through a strange encounter many years ago. Two anxious villagers brought a boy to my clinic with the embarrassed statement: 'There's something wrong with him.'

The boy himself looked angry, but said nothing.

No further history was forthcoming.

The boy was completely healthy, and I was completely foxed.

Finally, they sent the boy out, and confronted me with vehemence. Hadn't I noticed *the boy had no testicles*?

I contradicted.

They clarified.

Yes, they knew the boy had testicles, but at his age, they should be twenty times as big! If this got about in their village, it would bring them great shame. In their family, they were all real men.

Up went their dhotis to prove the point.

Both men, father and uncle, had huge filarial hydroceles.

'Standard size,' they said modestly.

Naturally, they expected more of their sons.

So, who sets the norm?

In July 2017, the *New England Journal of Medicine* published a study: 'Health Effects of Overweight and Obesity in 195 Countries over 25 years'.* The contents, meant to startle the planet into action, left me underwhelmed.

The paper held this cogent data:

In 2015, a high Body Mass Index (BMI) contributed to 4 million deaths, which is 7.1 per cent of deaths from any cause. And, 39 per cent of these deaths occurred in people with a BMI less than 30.

2.7 million of these 4 million deaths were due to 'cardiovascular illnesses'.

Diabetes contributed to 0.6 million deaths.

If you were to look at these figures solely from the Indian viewpoint, you would, like me, be baffled.

BMI or Body Mass Index is the international standard for gauging obesity, despite the obvious difference between Asian, European and African body structures.†

The international BMI cut-off for *overweight* is 25.

In India, where the problem is overwhelming, the need for a different parameter has long been expressed, but no change has been enforced.

I regard a BMI cut-off at 23 as more befitting our population.

The international BMI value for *obesity* is 29 or more. Any Indian with a BMI over 25 should be considered obese.

*An analysis of data from 68.5 million persons to assess the trends in the prevalence of overweight and obesity among children and adults between 1980 and 2015.

†We'll talk more about this in the chapter 'Measuring the Body'.

We are much fatter, and much sicker, than the West.

Our fatter and sicker people are much younger.

The global problem needs to be customized to your life and mine.

That, in a word, is what is lacking in our perception of the Big O.

For the past decade, I have looked at the problem from this context, and this book records some observations in answer to the question: *What are the drivers for obesity in India?*

Perhaps I had better explain the term 'driver' here.

When an epidemic emerges in a population, a number of factors contribute to the emergence of disease, to break the peaceful co-existence of 'pathogen' and 'host'. These pressurizing factors are termed 'drivers'.

This is easily understood in the emergence of infectious diseases. It doesn't take much imagination to see how an overflowing dump next to a fish market can set off an outbreak of typhoid or cholera. When it comes to non-infectious diseases, the connection is not so obvious. But the environment contributes even more closely to non-infectious diseases.

Ask anyone who has seen or experienced an illness in a new environment, and you will find they have a ready explanation for it.

Hawa badal gayi hai is a common bhasha colloquialism.

That is street cred for environmental change.

Because an element of personal choice enters the question, many of these non-infectious diseases are dubbed 'life-style diseases'.

Obesity seems non-infectious and non-communicable only because that is the unchallenged view at present. Look around you, and you will see clusters of obese men and women in closed groups—not necessarily related. In families, of course. But in offices too.

The immediate explanation is obvious, the same set of factors are influencing them.

When an explanation isn't obvious, we shrug off the matter as 'genetic'.

Incredible, the amount of junk science we borrow for these generalizations, but as with all generalizations, there is a central kernel of truth.

'Hawa badal gayi hai' is a phrase that sums up a lot of observations on India's obesity explosion. The immediate picture it evokes is one of migration. A new place, a new life. And that, in a word, explains our dilemma.

Migrations.

Arrivals.

And the memory of departures.

And what does migration have to do with obesity?

Hawa kaise badalti hai?

Ibn-e-Batuta, pehenke joota, chal pada toofan mein...

Sarveshwar Dayal Saxena's poem is about every Indian today. We are all travellers as intrepid as Batuta, and as eager to absorb the landscape wherever we pitch our tents.

What? You've never travelled, and yet—

Hold on, let me redefine *migration.*

To go from one place and settle in another need not always mean you leave your city to live in another, although this is the common impression.

That is only the third most common sort of migration.

The commonest?

The migration from home to school or office.

And the second commonest?

The migration into virtual reality.

You could begin by arguing that Indians have always been migrants, and we never were obese till now. We (men, mostly) have always worked away from home since time immemorial.

Here is where I differ. I have a real problem with these mists of antiquity.

Human memory does not stretch that far.

We can take a look at the last 200 years.

Seriously, let us do that.

Take a look at life in British India. *Indian* life in British India. And you'll wish you hadn't.

The commonest lifestyle disease then was starvation as we teetered between epidemics and famines.

Hunger and Disease are no respecter of persons.

So what if your ancestors were exalted personages? Chances are they did not live long enough to explore any of today's lifestyle diseases.

Migrations *within* India occurred throughout the nineteenth century for much the same reason they occur today—in search of food, employment, a better life.

Why should the fallout be any different today?

Looking at a day in office as a migration does not require a leap of faith.

The commute is arduous. Breakfast, if there was one, is a rapidly vanishing memory by the time you clock in. In some cases you go from a noisy and beleaguered environment into a cooler, calmer one. In many more cases, one form of mayhem is simply exchanged for another.

Either way, it takes a while to get into the groove.

The effort of that puts a damper on body signals.

Physical discomforts—a straining bladder, hunger, exhaustion—have to be ignored in order to get on with the job.

When, finally, there is a let up, there's the tussle between the dabba packed at home by loving hands, and the savoury scents floating in from the street. Most often, the dabba wins.

And that is even more tragic.

Yes! I felt that!

Your acute disapproval.

Your disapproval is evident. Let me explain. Between duty and desire I stand firmly by duty, just not blindly. Sure, that dabba is overflowing with love. But what *else*?

No matter what the contents, is the dabba meal enough to stave off hunger till your dinner at 9 p.m.?

Of course it isn't.

Realistically, one should eat again about four hours after lunch, and if you don't, won't or can't, there will be endless cups of tea.

The trip home is even more fraught. I can speak for my city.

Churchgate Station is the capital of glut at going-home time. Forget our coffee, bananas and biscuits past. Amchi Mumbai won't be seen dead eating a vada sambar or Punjabi samosa now. Everything edible is Chinese, Thai, or Italian. Speak not of breads but of waffles, burgers, wraps, rolls, puffs and patties. Everything is so conveniently packaged. Even a turd will make a delectable snack, if shrink-wrapped.

Who doesn't want a snack at that hour? Lunch is a dim memory, and dinner is still miles away.

'So hygienic! You can be certain you won't catch anything. This isn't raaste ka maal in a newspaper cone.'

'Served so decently in aluminium foil, cling-film, Styrofoam. And, they always provide tissues.'

'Hot and fresh, what more can you ask for?'

'It isn't deep fried, there's no oil at all.'

'Good value! Really fills you for the price.'

And there's the swindle.

Hygienic is any snack in disposable wrappings.

Hot and fresh is yesterday's leftovers, microwaved.

That last argument, though, is absolutely flawless.

The snack sits in the stomach like cement. Because, for it

to survive all that packaging without turning limp and sour, it needs a helluva lot of fat and sugars. The packaging just raised the food value by 100 calories, probably more.

Sure, it isn't deep fried.

Even if baked, it still is a walking coronary. That dry flaky pastry encasement has enough fat to make a deep-fried samosa look like a sanyasi.

This is just us commuters at the end of a hard day, and god knows we need some energy to work our way home through the seven o'clock traffic once we get off that train.

Detour now and walk into a coffee shop.

Most of the customers here are regulars at that gym round the corner. They just drop by here between work-outs. They do not caffeinate. They opt instead for 'healthy' smoothies and wholegrain cookies—which earns them enough Brownie points to pig out on chocolate cake later.

Chocolate is good for you, everyone knows that, and that delicious double Dutch truffle is so light! Just air with a bit of cream.

Sure. One wedge has enough calories for a family of four to lunch on.

You could argue that a bare 20 per cent of commuters snack on their way home, and a minimal 10 per cent indulge in baked goods. The rest grow obese on ghar ka khana.

Shouldn't this be enough to tell us that we are bursting our belts because of the food we eat?

'Ghar ka khana', no matter which corner of the subcontinent you come from, is the holiest of holies, the one constant in a changing universe, the standard of perfection nothing can ever challenge or impeach.

Oh yeah?

Look at it this way. We are a nation divided by food: food rules, food prejudices, food inhibitions and food proscription EVEN BEFORE we countenance the shameful and persistent barriers raised by caste and creed.

At its most innocuous, this attitude is no more than a preference for taste and flavouring. A visiting child may refuse a familiar food and gravely explain, 'It tastes different at home.'

I like to remind myself of this when faced with near-impossible instances of prejudice, and the unbridled violence that accompanies it.

The horrifying story of Mohammad Akhlaq qualifies as national shame, but there are less public instances all around us. The principal of a large school in a Mumbai suburb once related this heart-rending tale.

The students in the primary school were from three large nearby slums. Like all inner-city children, they were hungry and undernourished. The school arranged for a reputable kitchen to provide a free lunch.

'The lunch was really delicious,' she told me sadly, and went on to itemize it—a different kind of khichdi every day of the week, chhole or ragda, and a sweet.

I knew the kitchen and had tasted the food, so I could vouch for hygiene, taste and nutrition.

'On the first day, all the children enjoyed the food. From the next day, not one child would touch the meal. Worried, we sampled the food, but there was nothing wrong with it. This went on for a week. They would simply stare at the lunch till we were forced to take the plates away. The children hadn't brought dabbas either, and we had to get bananas and biscuits. They had to eat *something*! I sent for the parents, thinking perhaps they didn't know what was happening. To my surprise all the parents told me they had instructed their children not to touch the food. "Who knows what's there in that food? Where has it come from? Who made it? Why is it free? We are not beggars—" These were just some of their reactions.'

'Irritated, I asked them why they hadn't sent dabbas in that case,' my friend continued.

'The answer was even more mystifying. "We told them it was wrong to eat the food. We gave them money. They could buy something if they wanted."'

If they wanted?

Those children were six years old. They had left their homes at 7 a.m. without breakfast. They would return home at 2 p.m.

And yet, the fear of parental disapproval had swamped the tidal surge of hunger in these little ones.

Not just their growing bodies, but their minds had been warped irretrievably by now.

Is this tomorrow's India?

'What did you do?' I asked.

'What *could* I do? I cancelled the contract. They went back to eating their dabbas, chips or biscuits usually. Or, they bought stuff at the gate. Horrible stuff.'

Bitter tears ran down my friend's angry face. There was nothing I could say to console her.

This, in the nation's most pluralistic metropolis.

Hatred and suspicion envenom us so deeply, that paranoia is India's most prevalent disease. It contributes in many subtle ways to all the body's other griefs—including obesity.

Discounting the paranoia of hate, if we were to read food prejudice as a child's forthright comment, 'Your food tastes different from mine,' it leads up to many interesting questions.

Three households on the same street may cook the same dish, and yet each will have a distinctive taste.

So why is my upma different from yours?

That is the question that started off my enquiry ten years ago, irritated by the 'diet sheet' common in hospitals: *One serving of upma: 100 gm.*

'That doesn't tell me what's in the upma,' I pointed out.

My protest made no sense to the nutritionist. 'Upma is rava,' she frowned.

'Yes, but how do you *make* it?'

That earned me a shrug. Clearly, she was above such frivolities.

So I readdressed the question to myself, and got busy.

Food is all about nutrition, but eating it is all about taste and satisfaction. Let us see how the two merge together in a perfect meal.

The Perfect Meal

By definition, a good meal is one that is planned with science, cooked with intelligence and care, served with love, greeted with appetite, tasted with pleasure, and eaten with respect.

Or—

A good meal is one that smells good, tastes good, and feels good afterwards.

Much the same thing.

All that makes it smell good, taste good, and feel good afterwards is—science.

The science of food is pretty simple. There are three food groups, and we need to eat all three.

The three groups are: Carbohydrates, Proteins and Fats.

Periodically, one of them is criminalized, and we're bombarded with dire warnings for a while.

Under attack presently?

Carbohydrates, or 'carbs', as they're slightingly called today.

Needless to say, these condemnations are always issued from richer nations.

By now everyone knows that the Third World gluts on carbs.

The First World prefers proteins and saturated fats.

This twenty-first-century belief is nothing less than a violent imposition of caste, the declaration of a New World Order.

Again, needless to say, such pronouncements are either junk science or misreadings of good science.

To stay alive, we need all three—fats, carbohydrates and proteins.

In the language of a primary school textbook, carbohydrates are energy fuel, proteins are body builders, and fats take care of body temperature, hormones, and, oh yes, the brain.

Those are just words. Besides, unless we enquire into the matter, we're clueless about what proteins, carbohydrates and fats do within the body.

How do we recognize them?

What do they look like, smell like, taste like?

How do we find them in the foods we eat?

Walk into the kitchen and sort out the basics.

CARBOHYDRATES are often called 'sugars' in discussions about food.

Sugar, granulated sugar, icing sugar, Demerara, brown, jaggery,* honey—are all carbohydrates.

But so are less sweet staples: all grain, milled or whole. This includes the entire gamut of cereals in your kitchen and also in the new faddy 'health food' stores. AND their flours. Here is a quick headcount:

Wheat: This includes atta, maida, daliya. BUT ALSO: sooji (rava), pasta, seviyan.

When you think maida, think anything baked: breads, cakes, biscuits, cookies.

Rice: All the different kinds of rice you can think of. AND puffed rice, beaten rice, red, black, and purple rice, rice from anywhere in the world.

Millets: India has a variety of regional millets that are slowly crossing borders. These are the commonest: sorghum

*Jaggery is a Portuguese corruption of the Sanskrit '*sharkara*'—brown lumps of condensed sugarcane juice, also called gur.

(jowar), spiked millet (bajri, kambu), finger millet (nachani, ragi), foxtail millet (tenai), little millet (kutki, samai), kodo millet (kodon, varagu), common millet (chena, pani varagu), barnyard millet (sanwa, kuthiravolly).

Chances are that your kitchen may have a few of them. If not, check out the nearest supermarket, and get to know them.

Daals: Any, and, all of them.

What? Did you say protein?

Yes, you're right, but daals pack a hefty dose of carbohydrate too. A pulse is just a daal with its jacket on, and we have a cornucopia of pulses, count them all in.

Roots and tubers: These are plant larders of energy.

The ubiquitous potato, king of the kitchen, is a wonderful source of energy.

We also have more venerable tubers: colocasia (arvi), and a fine array of yams.

Root vegetables, like carrots and turnips.

Regional specialities, like tapioca, are carbohydrate concentrates.

Fruits: The sweeter they are, the more carbohydrates they contain, is a fair rule.

Bananas, all the zillion varieties that abound, are life-savers.

All carbohydrates are. They provide instant energy.

Deadbeat and miserable? Unzip a banana. Works every time.

Starch is a complex carbohydrate made up by linking together simple sugars. Most sweet-tasting sugars are disaccharides, made up of two linked molecules.

PROTEINS are body-building stuff.

And that doesn't mean just those bulging triceps, pushy pecs, and six-pack abs the gym promises you.

Proteins structure practically all body tissues, but they're so much more than masonry.

All the active processes in the body are powered by enzymes, and all enzymes are proteins.

When the diet is deficient in protein, we are just *weak*.

That said, where do we get this magic stuff from?

India is predominantly vegetarian. Even those who eat meat and fish seldom do so every day. So where do we look for vegetable sources of protein?

Daals and their jacketed forbears, pulses. These are legumes, the cotyledons of seeds meant to nourish the embryo plant. Daals supply most of India's protein needs, so their quality, availability, and digestibility, determine how effectively they nourish us.

Cereals also contain protein.

Seeds are meant to store nutrition for a long period. They are, of necessity, hard, and yield their nutrients with difficulty, as every cook knows. Most of them need to be soaked. Cooking time is long.

And, they're not always easily digestible—a situation the country at large calls GAS.

We have developed traditional ways of getting around these problems: soaking, grinding, fermenting, and adding a bouquet of aromatic spices that encourage digestive enzymes.

Proteins from **animal sources** are easier for the body to handle—simply because we evolved to digest them. They are also 'complete' proteins, containing all the essential amino-acids. Unlike plant proteins, animal proteins yield their nutrients more easily.

Professed vegetarianism should exclude all animal products, but what would Indian food be without dairy?

Dairy products, milk and curds, are our principal source of complete protein.

All dairy products have their protein yoked to fat.

Thick buffalo milk only has 3.1 gm of protein/100 ml, but the fat content is between 6–8gm/100ml.

Milk also is rich in carbohydrates.

(The other 'luxury' dairy products—cheese, paneer, etc. are better considered with the next food group.)

Our national distaste for **eggs** is simply tragic.

Eggs are as 'vegetarian' as milk.

The eggs in the market are all unfertilized and there is no question of accidentally swallowing the unborn.

An egg a day can get Indian children smiling in no time.

But that is an argument that will have no takers. In India, children are expendable.

All Indian children (yours excepted) are protein-deprived.

Egg protein is the gold standard.

All other proteins are measured against it.

Egg white is pure albumin and the much maligned yolk is a phospholipid, brain stuff.

Meat and fish deliver complete protein easily: a little goes a long way.

What about red meat and white? All flesh from mammals is nutritionally 'red' because of the muscle pigment myoglobin. 'White' meat—from chicken and fish has less of this pigment.

Proteins are large molecules made up of components called amino acids. Unlike sugars, amino acids contain nitrogen. Some of them also contain sulphur.

Twenty amino-acids are known to be proteinogenic, that is, they make proteins—and of these nine **cannot** be manufactured by the body, **and must be present in our diet.**

These *essential* amino acids are—isoleucine, leucine, isoleucine lysine, methionine, phenylalanine, threonine, tryptophan and valine.

Children also need some of the others that the adult body synthesizes.

'Incomplete' proteins are those which lack one, or more, essential amino acids, and most plant proteins are incomplete.

But trust us to have tricked our way out of this.

In India, everything is rice and daal—when it is not roti and daal. These combinations work for a very cogent reason. Daals are deficient in the amino acid methionine that cereals have in plenty. Conversely, daals are rich in lysine which is low in cereals. So the supremely satisfying combination delivers a meal with a complete amino acid profile.

FATS—instantly identified as a cooking medium in the kitchen—oil, margarine or vanaspati, butter, ghee.

Fats fall into two large groups: saturated and unsaturated.

Saturated fats are solid at room temperature on a cool day.

Unsaturated fats are liquid—**oils.**

(Because of a difference in chemical structure, coconut oil solidifies easily on a cool day.)

In addition to these obvious sources of fat, there are many others, some covert, some simply overlooked.

Nuts, delicacies de luxe, can't possibly be gobs of fat, can they? But that's exactly what they are. An almond is 50 per cent fat.

That reeks of heresy. How can the incomparable badam, the very repository of perfection, be dismissed as fat? And the walnut, the aromatic heart of dark and delectable patisserie, that too?

Yes.

But, who ever said fat is bad for you?

So is your kitchen covered?

What about the one group I have neglected to mention, the green life-blood of Indian cuisine, vegetables? Where do they fit in?

Vegetables are mainly cellulose—a complex indigestible carbohydrate. Think of it as elegant and effective packaging for—water.

Vegetables are nearly all water, even the ones that don't appear to be so.

The life-blood of vegetarian India is just—water?

Yes, but also carbohydrate, some protein, a jot of fat, minerals, vitamins. All good stuff, trust me.

Now that we've seen what food is all about, how much energy do your meals provide through the day?

Simply staying alive requires a lot of energy. That is the Resting Energy Expenditure (REE), easily calculated from a simple formula.

For men: REE = 900 +10 x wt in kg

For women: REE = 700 +7 x wt in kg

Naturally, that is hardly enough to keep up with our busy lives.

Sedentary, moderately active, and very active people require their REE multiplied by factors of 1.2, 1.4 and 1.8.

That is between 1,500 and 2,500 calories a day—if you are in good health and not stressed out. If not, you need more.

That is a lot of energy.

So let us see how much of energy each food group offers.

One gm of carbohydrate yields 4 calories, one of protein the same, but 1 gm of fat yields 9 calories.

The standard recommended energy intake from each food group is:

45–60 per cent from carbohydrates

10–15 per cent from protein

When it comes to fat, the recommendation is up to 30 per cent

Work it out. That is an unconscionable amount of oil.

The ICMR* guidelines for 2011 state, confusingly:

> The total fat (visible + invisible) in the diet should provide between 20-30 per cent of total calories. The visible fat intake in the diets can go up to 50g/person/day based on the level of physical activity and physiological status. Adults with sedentary lifestyle should consume about 25g of visible fat, while individuals involved in hard physical work require 30-40g of visible fat. Visible fat intake should be increased during pregnancy and lactation to 30g.

Really?

Now, let's get lunch going.

Ordinary ghar ka khana, comfortable servings. Rice, daal, vegetables. Dahi as an add on, perhaps. Maybe two sorts of sabzi. A pappadam. Pickle. Add all this up and it will top at a modest 350 calories. This, you'll agree, is what most of us eat every day.

To most Indians, this describes the perfect meal.

How did this perfect meal make us so fat?

*The Indian Council of Medical Research (ICMR) is responsible for the formulation, coordination and promotion of biomedical research, and it is one of the oldest and largest medical research organizations in the world.

Measuring the Body

Are we, truly, as fat as we're made out to be?

The FAO* (Food and Agriculture Organization of the United Nations) report for 2017 says 190.5 million Indians are undernourished. That is probably an underestimate.

25 lakh Indians die of hunger and hunger-related causes every year.

Dare we call ourselves *fat*?

In 1975, India had 0.4 million obese men and 0.8 million obese women.

In 2014, these figures have altered out of all recognition—9.8 million men, and a staggering 20 million women. Among women, the severely obese number 3.7 million.

The trouble with statistics is that it distances the issue.

...they are as sick that surfeit with too much as they that starve with nothing was Shakespeare's wry comment in 1605.

In our India of 2018, we need neither reports nor statistics. The paradox eyeballs us on every street.

Every morning, a short walk takes me past six schools and a college before I reach the city's lowest common denominator, the railway station. This gives me a fair random sample of the city's population. And this is what I see.

---

*The Food and Agriculture Organization is an agency of the United Nations that addresses international efforts to defeat hunger. Its motto, *Fiat panis* is Latin for 'Let there be bread'.

Children from the municipal schools are stick-legged and undernourished. Their accompanying parents (mothers mostly) are young, fit and harried.

Two private schools on the next road have kids of the same size—but only till puberty. Adolescents in these schools look very different. Each group has at least two who are large, pale and puffy, with accompanying moms built to scale.

Air-conditioned buses offload children at the International School. Even the eight-year-olds here are large.

Outside the college, young men and women swarm the carts of the Khao Gali. Not yet 9 a.m., but most have the bleary look of having spent long hungry hours. They probably left home without breakfast, to make the 8 a.m. lecture, but even the fed look worryingly tired.

College couture leaves very little to the imagination, and almost every young man and woman has a cushiony collop at the waist.

By the time I get to the station, I'm part of a humungous bolster of fat on the move. Almost everyone has a paunch so tense it looks muscular.

Women, scarcely into their thirties, carry compacted slabs of cellulite vacuum-packed in lycra and hosiery. Sari wearers are more disinhibited: midriffs rise like idli dough, bulge and overflow. The prevalent style in shalwar qameez leaves a flap hanging dismally between upholstered bulwarks of haunch and thigh.

Men, lacking the pizzaz of enhanced couture, simply loom massive in misery. And that's just the young.

Men and women my age don't give a damn. Perspiring, plethoric, grim-faced, we plod on, out of breath, hips and knees and spine in varying degrees of decrepitude. People no longer stride. The middle-aged either list or waddle.

The old are much jauntier: their limbs pack titanium, guaranteed indestructible, unlike bone and cartilage.

But that is still *other people*. To view the situation against one's own context literally means measuring oneself.

Body Mass Index is the standard assessment of body size. BMI calculators are accessed at the touch of the keyboard, and you can have your value within seconds. The internationally accepted grouping is:

BMI <18	underweight,
18–25	normal weight
25–29	overweight
29	and over is obese.

Neat, but its accuracy in conveying the idea of 'harmful' fat was questioned as far back as 1947, when a French physician, Jean Vague of Marseilles, made a very specific comment on the complications of obesity. What mattered, he said with no vagueness at all, was, *where*, and not *how much*. He pointed out that abdominal obesity was linked with disastrous events, lower-body obesity was not.

In 1947, nobody cared a whit.

In the 1980s, forty years later, Vague's ideas were echoed by other observers. Abdominal obesity was strongly correlated with bigger problems—heart attacks, strokes, diabetes.

BMI doesn't tell us *what is* being assessed. A flabby businessman and a muscled athlete may have the same reading. In the businessman fat is being assessed, in the athlete it is muscle. BMI also doesn't tell us *where* the fat is, or indeed if there is an accumulation of fat at all.

If that last thought gave you pause, the next time you're in a crowd, do a quick paunch count.

Paunches vary, of course, from the frankly globular to the modest bump above the belt or the wobble in the T-shirt.

Count them all, and every time you spot one, ask yourself: *Is this person fat?*

You'll be shocked to discover how often the answer is: *Good heavens, no!*

To put it baldly, a person of normal weight may have a more than noticeable paunch. He or she may also have a 'normal' BMI.

Another situation where the BMI is a poor indicator is in children in whom growth has to be factored in, and BMI has no age correlation.

Despite all these drawbacks, we still rely slavishly on BMI.

It doesn't matter so much if you're Caucasian, as this index then fits better.

White Americans dutifully keep to cardiovascular normalcy within the 'healthy' range of BMI.

But Asian-Americans seem poor respecters of BMI norms.

Around the time that abdominal obesity was acquiring a tie-up with cardiovascular illnesses, it became evident that Asian-Americans were prone to heart attacks at a much lower BMI.

That was twenty-five years ago.

In India, we are still using the international European standard BMI to evaluate ourselves. We read ourselves through Western eyes, and that is really dumb when all the evidence is out here on our streets that despite all our fairness creams, blonde hair colouring, and coloured contact lenses, we do not look European.

In popular perception, BMI is still the standard.

In medical perception, concerned physicians have rebelled vociferously, but have largely gone unheard, not just by the public but by their own colleagues as well.

A cut-off point of 23 instead of 25 has been urged. A BMI above that should be considered overweight. I have consistently adopted this, but I do not rely on BMI as a satisfactory index.

Based on BMI, only 13 per cent of Indian adults are obese as against the staggering figure for Americans, 39.8 per cent. But Indians within this 'safe' BMI range are prone to all the complications of obesity. Even more alarmingly, the worldwide trends in obesity, published in *The Lancet* of 10 October 2017, show that although obesity in children of high-income countries appears to have plateaued, children in middle-income countries, especially in Asia, continue to grow progressively obese.

Time then, if not for today, but for tomorrow's India, to abandon this mismeasure of obesity.

Jean Vague's idea was published the year we became an independent nation. Let me trace Vague's idea in parallel with our own changing profile.

Seventy years is a very long time, and it is very difficult for an Indian in his or her thirties to visualize life that far back, so let me choose a more proximate segment of time—the 1980s.

In 1985, prospective studies—the term describes a cohort observed through a period of time—showed abdominal obesity to be associated with increased risk for ischemic heart disease, stroke and death. This finding was not aligned to the total degree of obesity. Even limited abdominal obesity was identified as a major health risk.

The waist circumference was matched against hip circumference to judge abdominal obesity—the higher the ratio of waist to hip, the greater the cardiovascular risk.

Fifteen years later, a very large study, conducted over sixty-three countries, examined a very simple determinant, waist circumference, and related it to the presence of diabetes or cardiovascular disease. There was a definite correlation. A high waist circumference was associated with the presence of diabetes and cardiovascular disease at all levels of BMI, even in those who might pass for 'lean'.

These findings were replicated in other prospective studies.

One study also suggested that a 5 cm reduction in waist circumference could decrease cardiovascular risk by 11 per cent in men and 15 per cent in women.

There was an even more intriguing discovery. While an enlarging waist circumference increased cardiovascular risk, an expanding hip circumference (and lower-body obesity) was actually found to be protective.

Measuring risk became even more focussed with the knowledge that a raised waist circumference was linked with an abnormal level of blood fats. This observation also distinguished 'visceral obesity', or fat deposits within the abdominal cavity, as against the readily visible deposits beneath the skin.

Measuring waist circumference requires nothing more than a tape measure, but how do we measure fat deposits within the abdominal cavity?

Of course there is imaging. A CT scan, to begin with. But I am not talking machinery here. Between me and my mirror is just—air. How can I find out if my modest paunch is more worrisome than it appears?

The Sagittal Abdominal Diameter (fittingly shortened to the acronym SAD) is a dependable indicator of visceral fat.

It's easily assessed. Lie down on a flat surface, and balance a ruler on the peak of your tummy bulge. The vertical distance between the couch and the ruler is the bulge made by intra-abdominal fat.

But that's an assessment better left to your doctor. Assess yourself by measuring abdominal circumference.

For practical purposes, I find that measuring the maximum abdominal protrusion works best. This is literally how far your paunch sticks out. It's at a different level in everybody, and easily located, generally a little below the 'tailor's waist'.

The upper limit of 'normal' for men is 85 cm, for women 82 cm.

If you consider a 'tailor's waist measurement', reduce that by 2 cm to stay within 'normal' limits.

That's it, then.

If I have a BMI over 23, and a paunch that measures

more than 82 cm, and I'm Indian—I'm overweight, and obese is where I'm headed.

Now after we have that defined, how obese is our nation?

In a study done on 200 'apparently healthy workers' in Delhi, 54.5 per cent were obese and 17 per cent were overweight. Half of the sampled population had waist circumferences above acceptable limits.

Again—so what?

Few people will concede to being overweight until they actually tip the scales at OBESITY. At that point, a different argument takes over: *Love me, love my bulge*. From then on it is an endless whinge. Funny, because, it gets us right back to square one by making obesity something that we see.

But that isn't true.

The cosmetic challenges of obesity—bulge, wobble, jiggle, jounce, circumference, even tonnage—are mere irritations. We wouldn't think so, would we, from the vast industry devoted to their repair?

The serious aspect of obesity is elsewhere. It is invisible, until it announces itself as a disaster.

We have euphemisms for such disasters. We call them 'lifestyle illnesses'. Getting one places us among the privileged. It upgrades our shopping to an entirely new level. From celery and olive oil, Nikes and track pants, to spas for meditation and massage, bypass, transplant, immortality.

Living this out is tougher. The outrage of it begins to hit. This is illness, dammit. It is making me sick. It feels awful, I feel awful, and I'm long past caring how I look.

That is what obesity really is. It is walking around with twenty kilos permanently strapped on you, and perhaps ten of those are visible. But the concealed ten are silently, steadily, stealthily working their harm.

The Adipocyte at Home

Fat is good, and it is essential, right? Why then does it invite such opprobrium? What harm can something as beautiful and intelligent as fat possibly do?

Beautiful will pass without argument, but isn't *intelligent* a wee bit extravagant? Just because the brain is 60 per cent fat, does it necessarily follow that fat has a brain?

It all depends on how we look at it.

To medical undergraduates dissecting a cadaver, fat seems an unnecessary intrusion. It keeps the body from resembling the line diagram in the textbook. As a surgeon, one gets a different perspective. Suddenly, fat slams you with its vitality. Fat *bleeds.*

At this moment, the surgeon and the tissue are at odds. To the surgeon, fat seems needlessly squelchy. Why would a cushion of subcutaneous fat need so much blood?

Fat gets pumped with 3ml/100gm/*minute* when you wake up after a good night's sleep.

That isn't just breakfast. It is breakfast on the balcony, with WhatsApp.

Nutrients, oxygen and *news.*

Blood brings in gossip from the far corners of the body, and fat chatters right back.

If we were to eavesdrop on a layer of subcutaneous fat—condign, nice and plump, far from obese—the noise would be deafening. We would need a dragoman.* Some of those

---

*Dragoman is a corruption of the Arabic *tarjumaan*, translator.

cell signals are pure Greek. Endocrine, paracrine, juxtacrine, autocrine—the suffix comes from the Greek *krinein* for *separating*, for *sifting*.

Information is being sifted everywhere, and in fifty different sharps and flats. So many voices—and from so many unexpected cells.

Fat is just *fat*. Or is it?

Okay, I'll grant it blood vessels. But nerves?

Fat is simply twitchy with nerves.

It doesn't feel that way. It doesn't seem particularly sensitive, leave alone sentient. Pleasant, yes, but phlegmatic. That is because the nerves in fat are largely *autonomic*.

Our conscious and willing nervous system has a penumbra—the involuntary nervous system. Its other name is more revealing of its true nature. Apostate, maverick, rogue, wildcard, it has a mind of its own: the *autonomic* nervous system. It is a balance of two opposing forces. The *sympathetic* nerves (which have nothing to do with fellow-feeling) and the *parasympathetic* nerves make up the two divisions of involuntary control. Not only do they fine tune the concealed organs, but they also influence the crank and shaft of the body's crude machinery.

Sympathetic nerves secrete a chemical very like the one produced by the adrenal glands, so they're called *adrenergic* nerves. The other sort, parasympathetic, produce acetylcholine, but we'll pass on that for the nonce, because adipose tissue specializes only in adrenergic nerves.

Quite a lot of them nest around adipocytes, which means their chemical noradrenaline has a lot of say. Adipocytes have several sorts of adrenergic receptors, predominantly of the β (beta) sort, and they trigger off *lipolysis* or fat breakdown.

The flush of blood brings in the hormone insulin, famously associated with diabetes. Insulin encourages the adipocyte to make more fat and to store it. In the tug of war between the adrenergic nerves and insulin, the adipocyte would be perpetually conflicted if it didn't have a mind of its own.

Adipocytes produce chemicals of their own that act in every which way. They produce lipoprotein lipase which converts circulating lipoproteins into free fatty acids that easily cross the cell membrane. Another chemical decides how much of fat is taken in. The prime movers in lipolysis within the adipocyte are Hormone Sensitive Lipase, HSL (adrenergic-sensitive) and the adipocyte's own secretion, Adipose Triglyceride Lipase, ATGL. They have different points of action: ATGL breaks triglycerides into diacylgycerol and HSL converts them into monoacylglycerol. This calls for an enzyme to further break up monoacylglycerols into fatty acids and glycerol—and this enzyme, too, the adipocyte provides.

In addition, there is also perilipin, a chemical that unzips the membrane around the oil droplet, baring it for action.

Lipolysis takes place when energy demands are high: during fasting and during exercise, when adipose tissue sends out a rush of fatty acids for the muscles to use as energy by oxidation (think aerobic). This gets reversed by insulin in times of plenty and peace and quiet.

Evidently, the delicate sensor that decides our state of energy balance is—the adipocyte. The adipocyte manages this through a slew of chemicals it sends out into the circulation, its *endocrines*. There are quite a few of these. The most famous, of course, is leptin.

In 1994, Jeffrey Friedman, a molecular geneticist working on a mouse model of morbid obesity, isolated the *ob gene* and its product, leptin.

His pioneer paper modestly stated: 'The ob gene product may function as part of a signalling pathway from adipose tissue that acts to regulate the size of the body fat depot.'

Since then, *leptin* has entered common parlance.

I overheard, 'My leptin's given up on me' at a coffee shop recently, the speaker quite concealed behind a tipsy tower of chocolate cake.

Leptin, a hormone secreted by the adipocyte, is the STOP! signal to eating. It acts directly on the hypothalamus, as we shall see when we explore the mechanisms of appetite. But it is not merely an appetite controller. The adipocyte produces leptin in response to the amount of fat in the body. This takes the story in an entirely different direction. The adipocyte meters its output of leptin in keeping with the state of adiposity. *When we get fat, fat tells us to eat less.*

Does adipose tissue have an inbuilt obesity control?

Yes, it does, and leptin is just one of them.

In addition to reducing appetite and making us refuse dessert, leptin also urges every cell in the body to burn up fats.

Are obese people deficient in leptin?

Quite the opposite. Leptin levels rise in obesity, but the body has stopped listening. 'Leptin Resistance' is one of the determinants of obesity.

Adipocytes also secrete *adiponectin*. This is the anti-obesity hormone. Its sites of action are the muscle and the liver, and it makes these tissues very sensitive to the actions of insulin. It also increases the secretion of insulin from the pancreas. Adiponectin also acts on the adipocyte itself where it stops the breakdown of fat and increases the uptake of glucose. It has a cardio-protective effect, and prevents atherosclerosis by blocking inflammation.

If these virtues aren't enough, adiponectin also suppresses cancer cells. It is a gift that the adipocyte bestows on us. So much for adipose tissue being a health risk!

There is another hormone the adipocyte churns out. This one is downright dangerous! It is *resistin*, and it acts by—you guessed it—blocking insulin.

Besides these, new adipokines have been making the news every few months, constantly raising the adipocyte's clout. Without doubt, the adipocyte is crucial to normal metabolism.

Adipose tissue contains a surprising number of immune cells. Some are active in inflammation, others in the suppression of inflammation. All of them are known to secrete signalling molecules. In healthy and quiescent adipose tissue, they seem practically functionless. So why are they garrisoned here? Like a 'peacekeeping force', they are oxymorons.

Adipocytes in close contact with blood vessels secrete adipokines which diffuse through the wall of capillaries to exert a local effect. Most of the time, this lowers blood pressure.

Adipose tissue in contact with the heart and great vessels receives news about the state of oxidative stress on the heart muscle and responds by secreting protective adipokines.

The framework of adipose tissue, the extracellular space occupied by supporting cells, is also rich in lymphatic channels. Unlike blood vessels, these fine vessels are practically invisible because their contents are colourless. They are full of dietary fats, *chylomicrons*. Their local drainage sites are lymph nodes, congregations of lymphoid tissue rich in immune cells.

The lymph node is the local dump, where the debris of dead cells and vanquished pathogens is emptied. Immune printing takes place here, and starts off the secondary immune response to infection.

Adipose tissue in close proximity with lymph nodes is not just a passive onlooker. Its adipokines tutor and calibrate the immune response.

Within the adipocyte itself, mitochondria are the site of maximum activity. The breakdown and synthesis of fat requires a great deal of energy in the form of ATP, and this is produced within the mitochondria. The adipocyte is a canny sensor of the energy status of the body.

Just that thought is enough to catapult the adipocyte into the body's intelligentsia. Adipose tissue can no longer be considered a passive slab of flab, not even *before* it gets to be a slab of flab.

How does so smart a tissue become a slab of flab?

Energy excess is converted into more fat within the adipocyte. Under the influence of insulin, adipocytes manufacture triglycerides and stop exporting fatty acids into the circulation. Lipogenesis can start off from fatty acids and glucose to produce the intermediate compound Acetyl-Coenzyme A. Branched amino acids—valine, leucine, isoleucine—can also start off this process. *Thus, any dietary source of energy in excess of the body's demands can induce the adipocyte to increase its stores.*

A solitary adipocyte can only increase the size of its oil droplet to a finite limit. Every adipocyte in a fat depot can swell up and occupy more space. This requires serious tissue remodelling. If we need to shop for new clothes when we put on a few kilos, think of the restructuring necessary within the body to accommodate this recent change. What is happening within that bulge we have acquired?

Before we consider that, let us remind ourselves that adipose tissue behaves differently in its various depots. Here is a quick recap.

Skin fat has two compartments: the top layer (above the superficial fascia) is what is referred to as *subcutaneous* fat. It is metabolically different from the deep layer which is also white adipose tissue (WAT), but behaves more like visceral fat.

Subcutaneous fat is further classified as upper-body and lower-body. The second group is of great importance: Femoral fat refers to the collection of fat on the hips and thighs.

Visceral fat (VAT) is adipose tissue *within a body cavity.* Generally, this refers to the abdomen, and VAT has a completely different metabolic profile from subcutaneous fat. VAT is further distinguished by place names, but only two seem specially relevant: omental VAT and mesenteric VAT—this is fat on the two large abdominal membranes that support the important blood vessels of the stomach and intestine.

WAT has a number of preadipocytes or precursor cells in its architecture. Subcutaneous WAT, especially, femoral WAT has many more than VAT. These structural differences matter as adipocytes begin to store more fat.

With the onset of obesity, two principal changes are observed. Individual adipocytes grow bigger—they hypertrophy. The second change is in the resting population of immune cells. The inflammatory cells increase in number, in particular, macrophages, which assume a distinctive appearance.

The hypertrophied adipocytes show abnormalities, they secrete pro-inflammatory chemicals that block the action of insulin locally. The over-stuffed adipocytes finally die, and their debris further enhances inflammatory chemicals from the activated immune cells.

Meanwhile, the squeeze of bulging cells compresses and distances the nourishing capillaries, and creates a relative lack of oxygen. Hypoxia induces secretion of more inflammatory chemicals, all of which block the action of insulin. These inflammatory chemicals cause lipolysis, and fatty acids leak out of the over-burdened and dying adipocytes.

Local macrophages help clear some of this, but much of this inveigles its way into the circulation, and sets off the destructive phase of depositing fat in distant organs—principally the liver, pancreas and skeletal muscle. These organs are no strangers to fatty acids, but they lack the storage capacity of the adipocyte. The deposition of fatty acids is toxic to these organs. To begin with, it turns them resistant to insulin, so they can no longer utilize glucose for energy. As the situation worsens, their functions decline, and they undergo cell death by apoptosis.

Locally too, conditions worsen.

At first, inflammatory cells (macrophages) mop up some of the leaking fatty acids and cart away the remains of dead adipocytes. But these compensatory mechanisms are ineffectual in the face of the continuing energy excess. The tissue depot remodels itself by recruiting pre-adipocytes to fashion a new generation that can accommodate more fat. This is effective in only some depots. VAT doesn't make the cut. Subcutaneous femoral fat is a saviour—here more new adipocytes start swelling up, and draw in fatty acids from the circulation.

Lower body obesity, femoral fat, is considered protective. It lowers the free fatty acids in circulation, and prevents potential damage to the liver and cardiovascular system.

At other depots where the numbers of adipocytes cannot increase, the damage continues both locally and in distant organs.

This spatial restructuring calls for a new type of building material, collagen, which attracts even more inflammatory cells.

In VAT depots, the situation is awful, as preadipocytes are very few. The protective adipokines secreted here are now inadequate as adipocytes swell and die, and leak more and more fat into the circulation.

In going from a healthy, if overworked, tissue to an inflamed, hypoxic, debris-ridden slab of fat, adipose tissue has altered the energy balance of the body and introduced life-threatening complications.

The grim degree of insulin resistance and the high levels of circulating fat disrupt metabolism, and lead to illnesses that are diverse and apparently unconnected. To understand them better, they are all crowded under the umbrella term, Metabolic Syndrome.

Metabolic Syndrome

More than 20 per cent of Asian adults suffer from Metabolic Syndrome.

Metabolic Syndrome is a dangerous condition that carries a very high risk of diabetes mellitus and cardiovascular disease.

The disturbance in metabolism caused by obesity has a very wide fallout. It affects practically every bodily function, because every cell in the body is driven by the same basic metabolic processes.

Every cell (except those in the brain) needs insulin to convert glucose and fatty acids into energy.

Insulin is produced by the beta cells of the pancreas in response to a high sugar level in the blood.

The changes of growing obesity result in severe insulin resistance. This makes for a generalized energy crisis. All major body systems feel its impact. Some organs are especially vulnerable.

As glucose cannot now be utilized for energy, it accumulates in the blood. The pancreas, in response, pumps out more insulin.

As long as insulin has the upper hand, blood sugar levels will be maintained within normal range.

As obesity increases, insulin resistance also increases. This prolonged challenge to the pancreas eventually results in beta cell exhaustion, and precipitates diabetes.

This is Type II Diabetes Mellitus, as opposed to Type I Diabetes Mellitus which has an early onset and is not linked with central obesity.

90 per cent of diabetics worldwide have Type II diabetes. For the rest of this book, the diagnosis 'diabetes' applies to Type II diabetes only. This disease is what most Indians call diabetes, shakkar ki bimari, or more often simply, *sugar*, as in *mera sugar baddh gaya hai*. A statement that many, if not most, obese people will ultimately land up making.

Obesity disturbs the metabolism of sugar/glucose/ carbohydrate, call it what you will.

As fatty acids continue to leak out of over-burdened adipose tissue, insulin resistance increases, blood sugar rises, and the pancreas produces even more insulin.

In 1988, Gerald M. Reaven, of the Stanford University School of Medicine, described the link between high circulating levels of fats and high circulating levels of insulin. He pointed out that even a small increase in insulin can reduce the level of fats in the blood. Any situation where circulating fats increase will result in high insulin levels. If insulin resistance is so great as to prevent the action of the hormone, the level of fats in the blood will remain high. The liver will respond to this increased fat load by releasing glucose into the blood.

Reaven tested this chain of events in an animal model, and found them linked to the development of high blood pressure and cardiac problems. He concluded with this piece of wisdom:

> Based on these considerations the possibility is raised that resistance to insulin-stimulated glucose uptake and hyperinsulinemia are involved in the etiology and clinical course of three major related diseases—diabetes, hypertension, and cardiovascular disease.

That was three decades ago!

In India, where Metabolic Syndrome is rife, we seldom hear this diagnosis from our physicians. Which is a pity, because it can avert the popular impression that one can 'lose weight' simply by cutting out pakodas, taking a morning walk, and concluding it all with a glass of wheatgrass or karela juice at the park.

Before we embark on understanding the ravages of Metabolic Syndrome, consider what we're talking about when we talk about 'losing weight'.

'Weight' is a figure on the weighing scale—what does it tell me about what's happening inside me?

Suppose I'm five 5 feet 2 in height, and if the reading is 80 kg today and 78 kg a month later, should I cheer or take pause?

I would take pause to ask: I have lost 2 kg, but 2 kg of *what*?

Fat?

Water?

Lean mass?

By now, we know very well that these are vital considerations.

80 kg at 5'2" works out to a BMI of 32.2. Severely obese!

The metabolic changes brought about by obesity have upset the energy balance, so lean mass—principally, muscle—is at risk.

In health, more than 70 per cent of digested carbohydrate in the form of glucose is taken up by skeletal muscle. Here it is either used for energy, or is stored as glycogen. Resting muscle gets most of its energy from fats, through oxidation. During exercise, muscle switches fuels and opts, instead, for glucose.

When obesity sets in, muscle cells increase the 'transporter' chemicals which allow entry of fats into the cell. As fats accumulate inside muscle cells, the usual enzymes needed to oxidize them to form energy prove inadequate. As a result, this energy cycle is stalled and its by-products gather within the cell. These chemicals increase insulin resistance.

Muscle makes up 40 per cent of body weight. Imagine

the situation when nearly half your body's cells stop burning fat for energy. What happens to all that unused fuel? It keeps circulating, causing harm. Besides this, the accumulation of lipids within muscle cells and the generalized state of inflammation caused by obesity unleash widespread muscle destruction. Obesity leads to marked muscle loss.

Therefore, that 2-kg weight loss could very well be a 2-kg loss of muscle.

'Losing weight' is not synonymous with fat loss.

As we explore the state of the body in Metabolic Syndrome, it will become apparent that 'weight loss' is not the tipping point.

Then what is?

The waist circumference is the easiest way we can judge our own progress, so reach for that tape measure now.

As I mentioned earlier, few Indian doctors inform their patients of this diagnosis. Not only does this sustain the public delusion that obesity is a cosmetic problem, but, at an even more serious level, it transfers the onus of curing obesity on the patient.

The directive, 'Lose weight!' is frequently heard, but few doctors seem prepared to tell you how.

Metabolic Syndrome cannot be cured by will power or meta-magical fads and remedies. The household wisdom of those who love you is excellent moral support, and nothing more.

So, if you're obese, please consult an erudite doctor.

If your child is overweight, it is even more urgent that you consult a knowledgeable paediatrician.

How many obese people are diabetic?

In a study done across the country in thirty industrial communities ten years ago, more than 30 per cent of men and women had central obesity, and 10 per cent had diabetes.

More recent assessments are even more alarming.

A cross-sectional countrywide study of rural India in 2016 showed an incidence of 21 per cent for central obesity. Regionally, South India had the highest, 40 per cent, incidence of obesity. The mean incidence of diabetes was 9.5 per cent. Again, with a preponderance in the South. That is for the *rural* population. The figures for cities are much worse. And these are just statistics.

Obesity is, in itself, a pre-diabetic condition. Even if my 'sugar is normal', the high degree of insulin resistance speaks of a 'diabetes-like' situation which can easily slide into frank disease.

There is a small population of obese people who remain fat but fit. Curiously, they have large accumulations of femoral fat and not much of visceral fat. The jury is still out on whether this represents an ideal metabolic compensation.

Most obese people, though, either have or will soon get Metabolic Syndrome.

If you are an Indian man and your waist circumference exceeds 85 cm, or an Indian woman whose waist circumference exceeds 80 cm, you already have Metabolic Syndrome if you are positive for any two of the following three criteria:

a) high blood pressure
b) high blood sugar
c) excessive fats in your blood (high serum triglyceride, low HDL)

You need medical attention.

The common view of diabetes does not convey its dangers.

'High sugar' suggests that it is a condition easily remedied by cutting out sweets, and by 'controlling' it with a slew of drugs. What is left unsaid is that *diabetes damages every organ*. No part of the body remains untouched. Diabetes is a conduit to heart, brain, liver and kidney disease, to blindness, infertility and complicated pregnancies. Diabetes is not something you would wish even on your worst enemy.

A fasting blood sugar level of less than 120 mg/dl means you are not frankly diabetic. Anything over 100 mg/dl should get you worried.

What about high blood pressure? What is its special relationship with obesity?

More than 60 per cent of obese people have high blood pressure, hypertension.

I prefer the term high BP to hypertension for purely semantic reasons. All too often I've heard the word 'hypertension' being interpreted literally, as in 'When he's stressed out he goes, like totally, hypertensive.' A common answer nowadays to, 'Is there hypertension in your family?' is 'Oh yes, my family's hyper about everything.'

Among us Indians, hypertension is linked with a much lower BMI than Western data suggest. This correlates with our greater propensity for central obesity. I could have a 'normal weight' but a prosperous paunch would put me at risk for high blood pressure.

It gets worse. Obese people with high BP are more prone to cardiac problems than hypertensives who are not obese. And if this isn't enough, hypertension increases obesity.

Women particularly are at risk, especially young women. Before menopause, oestrogen has a protective effect on the heart and great vessels. With the onset of obesity, oestrogen is no longer so benevolent. In fact, obese young women are at a greater risk of developing hypertension than obese men of similar age.

The ways in which obesity raises blood pressure are many, commencing with the obvious mechanical challenge of sending blood across a larger network of vessels than existed before. This, in itself, increases the resistance against which the heart muscle has to pump. But there are more sophisticated ways in which adiposity tweaks the circulatory tree, beginning with the direct conversation between local fat and blood vessels, and the more injurious manipulation of kidney function.

The Renin-Angiotensin-Aldosterone system in the kidney is a delicate and temperamental hormonal determinant of blood pressure, and its critical balance is upset in obesity.

Obesity produces changes in the walls of blood vessels even before a rise in blood pressure manifests itself. One of the earliest changes is arterial stiffness. The vessel wall suffers changes in all its layers, all relatable to altered adipokines from obese fat depots. Insulin resistance, by itself, induces a rise in blood pressure.

As we learnt in the previous chapter, with the development of obesity, the adrenergic nerves are in overdrive. This increase of adrenergic chemicals is the body's equivalent of a Red Alert, and it places an added strain on the heart and circulatory tree.

Children, adolescents and young adults who are obese are at even greater risk of developing hypertension and cardiac problems. They deserve immediate medical attention rather than the usual parental optimism of 'Oh, he'll outgrow it.'

Dyslipidemia, or abnormal blood fats, is the third factor in Metabolic Syndrome, and ought to be the most self-evident. But it is, paradoxically, the most confusing.

What does 'abnormal blood fats' mean?

In laboratory language, it means an 'abnormal lipid profile'.

Twenty years ago, cholesterol was a familiar household bogey. The relationship verged on the affectionate. 'My cholesterol' had the same indulgence as a spoilt brat: to be controlled, but cherished nonetheless.

'My cholesterol' has grown up now, and its new avatars

are, confusingly, LDL, HDL, VLDL, apolipoproteins, triglycerides, and a whole lot of confusing ratios. Most labs provide kindly explanations in fine print.

When obesity tips over the limits of adipocyte expansion, triglycerides leak into the circulation. This shows up on the blood report.

HDL, (high density lipoproteins) and LDL, (low density lipoproteins) make up the good cop-bad cop cholesterol routine.

A lipoprotein is simply a packaged fat, bundled in a protein carrier for ease of transport. HDL totes away the excess of fats—triglycerides, cholesterol, phospholipids—from sites of potential harm, like the walls of blood vessels. It transports them to the liver which converts them into cholesterol that is secreted in bile.

That's right. The body *manufactures* cholesterol.

You don't get it simply from eating egg yolk.

The liver makes cholesterol in response to a high fat diet, secretes it into the intestine, then recycles most of it, back to the liver.

This recycling is done through a major vein which bridges the small intestine and the liver—the portal vein. This Entero-Hepatic Circulation may be of great importance in obesity, as bile acids regulate fat metabolism. Of late, it appears that they also regulate glucose metabolism. Add to these theories, the observation that visceral fat (VAT) increase is largely responsible for Metabolic Syndrome, and it does not seem a coincidence any more.

A chunk of adiposity surrounding the blood vessels that shunt absorbed food towards the liver must have a lot of say in the matter when you recall the various adipokines it secretes.

LDL, which packages many different kinds of fat, litters the body with its luggage. In particular, it offloads in the lining of blood vessels to set off that insidious evil—the atheroma or plaque. In no time at all inflammatory kinins set up a reaction that produces the clot familiar to us as a 'block'.

LDL's bad press is every whit deserved.

'Metabolic Syndrome' is a neat label that conveys nothing. It tells you not a damn thing about what it *feels* like.

Rita

Rita is having a good day.

The train spits her out on the platform a little too late to risk the ten-minute walk to her appointment. The stairs seem to go on and on, but she is out of the station at last.

Good to feel the cool fresh air after being cramped for half an hour! Good to get into a rickshaw, slide the bag off one's shoulder, slump in the seat and just—breathe. Bliss!

The driver catches her eye in the rear-view mirror.

'Tough morning?'

'Oh no, I'm having a great day.'

Rita has a list of mental boxes she ticks every day. Today she's ticked them all.

Morning walk. ✓

Karela juice. ✓

Vitamins. ✓

Calcium. ✓

Cup of matcha green tea. ✓

Spirulina tablets. ✓

Chia seeds. ✓

No snacking, except for a fistful of dried fruit and nuts Dinesh found at The Health Store.

Big bowl of yoghurt just before leaving home.

Packet of Marie biscuits on the train. Her last, from tomorrow she's going totally gluten-free.

Fudged the walk, but what the hell, who *walks* to an appointment with the orthopædic surgeon?

The lift attendant greets her like a familiar friend. 'Fourth floor?'

'No—'

'Ah, yes. Today is Tuesday. Second floor.'

'No. Fifth today.'

'Aisa? New doctor? Haddiwalla?'

She manages a polite nod and deflects the conversation. 'How are things with you?'

'Bas, thanks to good folk like you, everything is in running order.'

It is a slow lift. It lingers at the second floor, reminding her of last week's visit to the gynaecologist. It stops at the fourth for a minute as if by accident. She's only due to see the dermatologist next week for her allergies. And while she's there, she might as well get her hair fall looked at. Her hair looks just fine, but she's begun to *feel* bald with all the hair trails she leaves around the house. And Dinesh has been urging her to get her blood pressure checked.

Blood pressure? At her age? She's *thirty-six* for godssake! He won't say so, but she knows it is because she's so irritable. Wouldn't you be if you were so bloody tired all the time, and your knees were killing you, and you just wanted to sit down?

Of course she never feels tired when she's working. It is just these trips to one doctor after another that tire her out.

Even before she enters the clinic she knows exactly how it will go.

Two minutes across the table, another five putting her knees through the motions, a long list of tests, X-rays.

'MRI. X-rays don't tell you anything. Do an MRI,' the doctor says. 'Can't afford to neglect your knees. You'll need arthroscopy. We'll fix you up.'

'The pain is killing me.'

'Here you are then.'

Rita glances at the prescription. 'I'm taking all these tablets already, doctor!'

The doctor shrugs. 'You could try losing a bit of weight.'

Rita is fighting tears as she leaves. The lift guy maintains a sympathetic silence.

Dinesh calls just as she leaves the building.

'Same old, same old,' she answers.

'Did you get an appointment for an MRI?' he asks.

'Not yet.'

And she doesn't mean to. She's sick of the whole thing, this dream she's been chasing for two—no, three years, now. Who knew getting pregnant could be this difficult?

It carries a label now. PCOS. Polycystic Ovary Syndrome.

Dinesh has read everything on the net. He knows much more than the gynaecologist, and ends up irritating her.

He'll do the same this evening, Rita muses. They're seeing a physician at five, the gynaecologist thinks her thyroid might be the problem. Rita doesn't want to even ask what could be wrong with her thyroid. She doesn't want to think about it. It is just a word. She can't locate it in her body, and she doesn't want to.

It is now half half-past four.

Just enough time for a quick bite before she meets Dinesh.

Rita goes into the coffee shop across the road.

She hates coffee, but there is no other restaurant in sight. There still is the 'will power' box to tick, so she ignores the Dutch Truffle and ice cream and has a Peach Tea Cooler with a couple of cookies.

Dinesh is early. He rushes her through those X-rays, obtains an appointment for that MRI.

'Is it the thyroid?' they ask the physician in unison.

'Could be. We'll do some tests.'

'We did them last week.'

They show him the reports. He clucks sympathetically as he leafs through the folder.

'The tests are suggestive of hypothyroidism,' he says, and he prescribes thyroid hormone.

Her blood pressure is high.

'Not very,' the doctor says quickly, 'but it must be treated.'

Rita nods numbly through it all.

Dinesh leaves briefly and returns with the X-rays.

'Might as well get his opinion,' he mutters.

'Osteoporosis.' The doctor makes the word sound like a rare rich gift. 'I'll leave the tests to the orthopod,' he says, and prescribes Vitamin D.

'I'm taking that already!' Rita protests.

'Thank God it's the thyroid,' Dinesh says happily on the way home. 'Once you're on the hormone, everything will improve.'

They celebrate with a Chinese takeout meal.

Usually, it is Dinesh who sits up worrying, but he's fast asleep by the time Rita gets to bed tonight.

Rita takes her nightly dose of pills, fish oil capsules, and chyawanprash.

She sits awake a long while as she nurses her glass of haldi-doodh, thinking about what a good day it has been. Nonetheless, knowing no one can hear her now, she whispers into the dark, 'What if it isn't my thyroid?'

Rita's dilemma is shared by millions of Indians.

Like Rita, they've suffered from multiple ailments. They've been diagnosed with this or that illness, and not incorrectly. They've been medicated; and again, not incorrectly.

Like Rita, many obese women find it difficult to conceive. Some of them have Rita's diagnosis—PCOS.

Similarly, thyroid problems are quite common in obese people, particularly women. Very often this is 'subclinical hypothyroidism' where the patient shows no visible signs of thyroid deficiency, but blood tests reveal thyroid hormone abnormalities.

Like Rita, most of these patients are prescribed thyroxine as therapy.

The wisdom of treating a condition not experienced by the patient is always open to question.

Osteoporosis is well known in obese men and women with Metabolic Syndrome. The increased stresses on weight-bearing joints make them vulnerable to early wear-and-tear in obesity. Add to this the lack of physical exercise rife among the obese, and you get joint pains. The inflammatory profile of Metabolic Syndrome can set off arthritis. Bone and joint problems limit mobility and further compound obesity.

Depression is common among obese adolescents and young adults. To conclude this is merely because of poor self-image is simply facile.

As with all the other complications listed above, emotional and psychological changes can also be part of the biochemistry of Metabolic Syndrome.

So many illnesses, so many labels.

Doesn't it remind you of the parable of the six blind men encountering an elephant? Adi Shankara mentions it in the *Chandyoga Upanishad*, but I'll let the nineteenth-century poet John Gordon Saxe tell the tale:

It was six men of Indostan
To learning much inclined,
Who went to see the Elephant
(Though all of them were blind),
That each by observation
Might satisfy his mind

The First approached the Elephant,
And happening to fall
Against his broad and sturdy side,
At once began to bawl:
God bless me! but the Elephant
Is very like a wall!

The Second, feeling of the tusk,
Cried, Ho! what have we here
So very round and smooth and sharp?
To me 'tis mighty clear
This wonder of an Elephant
Is very like a spear!

The Third approached the animal,
And happening to take
The squirming trunk within his hands,
Thus boldly up and spake:
I see, quoth he, the Elephant
Is very like a snake!

The Fourth reached out an eager hand,
And felt about the knee.
What most this wondrous beast is like
Is mighty plain, quoth he;
'Tis clear enough the Elephant
Is very like a tree!

The Fifth, who chanced to touch the ear,
Said: Even the blindest man
Can tell what this resembles most;
Deny the fact who can
This marvel of an Elephant
Is very like a fan!?

The Sixth no sooner had begun
About the beast to grope,
Than, seizing on the swinging tail
That fell within his scope,
I see, quoth he, the Elephant
Is very like a rope!

And so these men of Indostan
Disputed loud and long,

Each in his own opinion
Exceeding stiff and strong,
Though each was partly in the right,
And all were in the wrong!

Moral:

So oft in theologic wars,
The disputants, I ween,
Rail on in utter ignorance
Of what each other mean,
And prate about an Elephant
Not one of them has seen!

In all these suffering victims, the elephant in the room, is Obesity. It is neither collateral nor coincident, but the gestalt in this growing variety of problems. Our blindness is largely because of a lack of understanding about the mechanism of the development of obesity.

We have looked at how obesity disrupts metabolism. But what sets off obesity?

In particular, why have Indians become, so suddenly, and so quickly, obese?

Yes, there is a Himalaya of surmise from researchers all over the world.

Animal models have been feverishly studied for decades.

Is obesity genetic?

Is it a reaction to some environmental toxin?

Why is it global?

Why is it no longer the disease of prosperity?

Why is India's rural population turning obese, even as there are starvation deaths among children?

Why are our children so obese?

Will they be diabetic and hypertensive before they are thirty? What will *their* children be like?

These are questions that concern each one of us, even those who aren't obese. And whatever answers research has to offer, all of them point to a common denominator: *food*.

Food isn't just about carbohydrates, fats and protein. It is about appetite, taste, relish and satisfaction, pleasures all of us consider central to health and well-being.

Dinner is just about ready. May I have the pleasure of your company?

Bon Appetit!

Tonight, dinner's a simple meal: daal, sabzi, roti, staples of half a billion Indian homes. An equal number substitute rice for roti. Either way, millions will be sharing the meal with us at this hour, so—bon appetit!

Deipnosophy—a complicated Greek word for a very Indian custom—is conversation around food, and usually not about food. While we chat, everything that happens within us is about food.

Deipnosophy isn't always the feast of reason and flow of soul it is expected to be within families. Home conversations are coded, intricate and intimate, pleasant and painful. We drag to the table all the burdens of the day, but within a few minutes, the leash slips. Grave issues give way to tease and laughter, voices lilt, stories begin...

Food is still ten minutes away, so what's happening?

The general loosening of the air has turned everything softer, and more welcoming, in the anticipation of pleasure. The sounds from the kitchen suggest the imminence of food, but something preceded that.

Aroma!

The scent of hot ghee, curry leaf, jeera came *before* the hiss of the garnish tempering the daal. It made us suddenly sentient, and not just of the meal. It alerted us to ourselves and our surroundings.

This is one of our more ancient truths. No matter what culture we belong to, eating together is a sign of amity and goodwill. Conversely, especially in caste-accursed India, eating apart is the worst form of 'othering'. Could this be more than cultural?

How can aroma change the emotional milieu?

Parfumiers among you are straining to answer that one, so let me restate the question. How can the aroma of food stimulate pleasure even before it stimulates appetite?

What is that complex accord of fragrances floating in from the kitchen?

The stream of odorant molecules is just a whiff to begin with. Unconsciously, we breathe deeper, drawing in more—if the aroma is specially delightful, this action becomes volitional. As the odorants enter the nasal cavity, they are captured by odorant receptors which translate them into electrical signals. Twigs of the olfactory nerves, charged with these signals, shoot off messages to the olfactory bulbs in the brain. From here it is a short trip to the olfactory cortex, and from there a swing to the orbito-frontal cortex—the thinking brain.

There is, also, a diversionary path which is more primitive—to the amygdala and the hypothalamus.

These older pathways explain our emotional response to aroma, the anticipatory pleasure which precedes the appearance of food, and also the way we apportion that pleasure.

It is easy to imagine our venerable ancestor, *Homo erectus,* the guy with the tool kit, calling over the family in the next cave to share his barbecue. But he bars the entrance to the fellow down the road whom he doesn't like. Too embarrassed to admit his dislike, he invents a pretty story: *us guys evolved from the brain of the Most High, those guys crawled out of his feet.* Very soon all guys from this end of the road won't eat with guys from that end, and before you can spell segregation, there is a caste system.

The tinkle and clatter from the kitchen, percussing this alaap of pleasure, is usually dampened by the stronger signal of smell. Still, auditory signals are pretty potent. I learnt this as a child of eight from Pooch, our cat.

Pooch was an exquisite, a startlingly beautiful tabby with a heart of stone. The only affection she ever showed was to things crisp and salty, with a marked preference for pappadam. Crisp flaky discs of pappadam were stored in an airtight tin that spoke directly to her glacial soul.

Pooch was a true gypsy, trailed by a long line of devoted toms, but no matter how far she ranged, she always heard the lid of the pappadam tin snap open. Within minutes in she flew through the kitchen window in a flash of gold. Just as quickly, she changed identity.

Metamorphosed, she bore no resemblance to the disdainful cat we knew. This was all kitten, arched back and throaty purr, velvet paws and melting eyes. Cupboard love, naked and unashamed.

It was gross, it was revolting.

And totally irresistible.

We simply surrendered that tin.

For a brief interval, all was crunch and crumble. Then, shaking the last flake of pappadam from her whiskers, Pooch swept past us with a sneer.

That pappadam tin didn't have a specially loud snap to it. Nobody else in the house heard it open. But that cat? It always could.

While I was telling you about the cat, an entirely different aroma distracted you.

The sweet scent of toasting wheat as phulkas balloon up makes us think not of roti, but of things more crisp and golden, and their arm-candy; delicate sophisticates, soft, sweet, creamy, decadent.

Advance information warns us to expect nothing more seductive than a roti, but imagination has supplied an entire alternate menu of festive delights.

Imagination is a lovely word, and elusive as perfume, but not that difficult to locate. In this case, the orbito-frontal cortex, the 'thinking' part of the olfactory pathway has located the scent of roti within its catalogue of flavours and placed it in the company of more festive delights. There is *association* here, relating odour to a familiar group of substances that offer the highest *reward*.

Reward, the 'feel-good' factor, is an evolutionary hand-me-down.

Foods that offer high energy are at a premium. The brain connects them immediately with appetite. They attract us even when we're not hungry. Foods high in sugar and fat get gold stars in the hypothalamus. When the odour of hot roti is the same as something much richer in fat and sugar, a jalebi, for instance, the hypothalamus semaphores a green light.

Here comes the food now.

The roti looks silken, the daal is molten gold.

The vegetables have retained shape and colour. Julienned carrots, spring peas, pearly onions, tender sprigs of cauliflower, tomato slivers: Kandinsky on a plate.

Everything on the table pleases in symmetry (unlike Hercule Poirot, I don't bemoan the absence of square eggs), and, I'm ready to eat.

Conversation stills to a pleasant silence as we touch the food. To most of us Indians, the use of cutlery is about as alien as making love with gloves on.

Children have a marvellous onomatopoeic vocabulary for food textures they dislike: *pach-pach, ishi-pishi, gluck, grrroo, kasha-kasha* ...

What do our fingertips have to do with appetite?

Again, textures, crisp, soft, creamy or firm, relate to high-energy foods with their feel-good reputation.

The slimy, gummy, rough and dry, are reminiscent of dangers our ancestors had to guard against: food that's decaying or desiccated. Rejection is almost immediate.

As with all hand-me-downs, this association too can play the devil with reason. The best protein in the world, an egg, is often rejected as slithery—*gluck*.

Our tactile signals to appetite don't stop at the fingertips.

As food brushes our lips, texture, temperature, and a stronger whiff of odour, all proclaim interconnectedness in the brain.

We continue to feel touch as food enters the mouth—touch as distinct from taste. The culinary world has a special term for this—mouthfeel. It is an index of *acceptability*.

Since we accept or reject foods based on this factor, why not take a closer look at mouthfeel?

Surprisingly, we overlook what happens to food once it enters the mouth. It changes, doesn't it?

Try chewing a flap of plain roti, and you'll feel it go from a pliant, faintly salty flatness to a sweet mush. Its aroma has intensified.

You can taste the surge of ghee in that small fragment, even if no more than a few drops had anointed the surface. Usually when roti is mere *delivery device* for more aggressively aromatic and spicy foods, we overlook its metamorphosis in the mouth.

Unlike magical metamorphoses, we can see this happen. (It is a mildly disgusting spectacle in the mirror, but watching it happen in another mouth, even your best beloved one, is Roald Dahl excess.) Some quick jaw work makes the teeth tear, crush, grind, and, with squirts of saliva, pulp and mash the roti.

The teeth are done now, but the mush stays on in the mouth, thoughtfully turned by the tongue, coated with juice.

By now every bit of pink in the mouth is a squelchy sponge of saliva. With all the expertise of a master boulanger the tongue kneads the food into a neat ball (more fashionably termed a *bolus*).

The Indian custom of kneading mashed rice into a soft

little ball before feeding a small child pre-empts this first phase. Sneak one of those from your little one's lunch some time—rice and daal with a dab of ghee, or rice and a creamy jot of curds—and you'll find it has the most sensuous mouthfeel.

The family apocrypha has the story of the Dog Doctor, circa early 1930s.

The Dog Doctor treated humans, but he had earned that label by having the healthiest children in the district.

It was a sprawling joint family, and there were about ten toddlers growing up together, sturdy little ruffians immune to the sniffles and runs that plagued other babies.

No surprise there, they were Doctor's kids, after all.

But my grandmother wasn't buying that.

'What do you feed them?' she asked, and his answer has earned him a place in lore: 'Oh, I just feed them like dogs.'

With a very young family of three of her own, my grandmother's outrage must have been visible.

'Come and watch,' he offered.

Here is what Grandmother saw.

The Dog Doctor's wife had somehow ended up being responsible for the entire crowd of infants, and he had devised this method for her relief.

A small empty room, grandly called 'the dining room', had been set aside for their meals. The Doctor cleaned it himself before every meal. He scrubbed the stone floor with boiling water, dried it with a bath towel, sprinkled some water as if to sanctify it—and made his exit.

Enter the Doctor's wife with two large bowls. One held balls of rice and daal, the other of curds and rice, standard toddler fare.

Before my grandmother's horrified eyes, she tossed the rice balls from the threshold into the room. Ten naked infants were air-lifted into the room, and sent on with a pat on their plump bottoms.

And then—the door was shut on them.

My grandmother's heart hammered with rage, but the other lady, with a beatific smile, invited her to share a tumbler of coffee in the courtyard.

Half an hour later, my grandmother, shaking with suppressed fury, followed her hostess to liberate the prisoners.

When the door was flung open not only was the floor clean, with not a squish, not a smear, not a leftover grain of rice in sight, but the ten toddlers were gurgling merrily, not a tear on their chubby cheeks.

'My little puppies,' the Doctor's wife said indulgently.

That Dog Doctor knew all about mouthfeel. My grandmother, though, never felt compelled to replicate his experiment.

Food oral processing is the clunky scientific label for this voluptuous sojourn of *feeling* food.

What exactly do we feel?

Bulk, suggestive of content.

Texture, perceptive of surface.

These perceptions relate to liquid foods too. A creamy soup and a sip of clear water have very different 'feels'.

Mouthfeel is dynamic, it alters as the food is chewed and rolled. In addition to changes in the mechanical structure of food as it is broken into smaller particles, there are chemical changes as well. The game changer here is saliva.

Spit, thook, ecchal is perceived as a contaminant in India.

There is the natural aversion to sharing body fluids with the next guy.

There is the educated dread of 'germs'.

And then there's something more, something so ancient that it has a place in the *Ramayana*, in the apocryphal story of Shabari. Rama and Lakshmana, wandering in search of Seeta, arrive at a hermitage on the banks of river Pampa. Shabari, an old ascetic, welcomes them and offers them the fruits of the forest—but in a most unexpected manner. She tastes each fruit before handing it to her guests. Lakshmana's indignation at the fruit being 'unclean' is sharply rebuked by Rama who insists that it is Shabari's act of devotion that makes her fruit the sweetest in the world.

I don't know when this legend entered the agglutinative epic. Valmiki, uttering the ur-text from the mists of antiquity, pictures Shabari offering fruit—but without tasting them first. Kambar's epic composition in Tamil from the twelfth century echoes this. Tulsidas in the *Ramcharitmanas*, 1576, ditto. I think it's telling that the legend should have entered the Ramayana discourse very recently.

Why did Lakshmana perceive Shabari's fruit as unclean?

Was it because Shabari was 'low born'? Unlikely, as she was introduced to the princes as the most spiritual and revered of ascetics.

More likely, Lakshmana shuddered at the thought of eating fruit glistening with someone else's saliva, entirely ignoring the spirit in which it was offered.

Rama's rebuke urges him to abjure prejudice.

The legend demands: *How can another's touch be pollution?*

A heart-rending cry, centuries before Ambedkar.

Shabari ke ber is one more of our beautiful truths being slaughtered in today's India. Only last week, a high-caste Thakurani killed a cleaning woman with her bare hands, bashing her head against a concrete wall for the crime of 'touching her bucket of water'.

In my redaction of the Shabari story, Rama spells it out more sternly. 'This is not about Shabari,' he clarifies, 'it is about saliva. Without saliva, no fruit ever tastes sweet.'

Without saliva, that roti will feel as abrasive as leather on the tongue. The teeth will render it more disgusting; it will now be coarse sand. Swallowing it will be difficult. It may even be dangerous. If the tongue propels that gritty debris into the throat, some of it may spill over into the windpipe.

Lubricated and emulsified, that morsel of roti can now be tasted.

The mashed up bolus tastes *sweet*. How can we explain *that?*

Roti is just atta and water. One doesn't expect wheat flour to be sweet unless it is tarted up.

But it is sweet, when you taste it. The magic is in the saliva. It contains a carbohydrate-breaking enzyme, salivary amylase, that cracks up the complex carbohydrate in wheat into simpler sugars.

The first stage of digesting dinner has actually begun much ahead of swallowing this first morsel of food.

Without this step, what taste would that piece of roti have?

We talk airily of tastebuds, making the tongue sound like a rosebush about to bloom. Tastebuds, or papillæ, make up the velvety pile of the tongue. There are three sorts of papillæ, circumvallate, fungiform and foliate, and we have to make do with just these to savour everything that enters the mouth.

Deep within these pappilæ are very specialized cells, the taste receptors.

Five tastes are universally acknowledged.

Sweet, salt, sour, bitter and umami.

The tongue is the body's fact-checker.

Salt? *Might be chemicals rich in sodium—watch out!*

Bitter? *Out before it kills you—that's poison!*

Sour? *Careful—that might be off!*

Umami? *Hmmm, good. Protein at last!*

Sweet? *Good stuff, pile it on!*

Unsurprisingly, we have more receptors for bitter than for any other taste, suggesting that taste developed as a gating mechanism to protect us from poisons in plants and spoiling food.

Sweet receptors are surrounded by a space enticingly

called the Venus Flytrap Domain. Sugars liberated by saliva enter this Domain. The Taste Receptor is activated. The presence of sugar is translated into a nerve impulse which is sent off to the Primary Taste Cortex in the brain which instantly recognizes this as 'reward food.' The reward circuitry—orbito-frontal cortex, caudate nucleus, amygdala, hypothalamus—is now active. This neural pathway releases the 'feel-good' chemical, dopamine.

Not all of us 'feel good' with the same amount of sugar. Some of us have receptors that seem to detect very low levels of sugar, and we just need less sugar in our tea.

What does this dopamine release in the brain achieve? Pleasure, certainly.

So is my roti simply mindless hedonism? For heaven's sake! That was just my first bite!

Dopamine translates pure pleasure into a logical command—*more!*

Another set of chemicals operating in parallel issues a statement of bliss. Opioids and endo-cannabinoids enhance pleasure.

Both reactions—wanting more of a delicious morsel, and the feeling of delight—drive appetite.

The region in the brain most actively involved in appetite and reward is the hypothalamus. One hypothalamic area in particular, the arcuate nucleus, is specially sensitive because the Blood Brain Barrier around it is weak, allowing hormones in the bloodstream direct access. It is a node for information from all parts of the body. Every nuance of metabolic change is perceived here. What better place to decide how much one should eat, and of what?

The arcuate nucleus has two sets of neurons. One set releases chemicals that increase appetite. The other does just the opposite.

The brain, despite its epicurean ideals of pure pleasure, can still empathize with the metabolic status, and blow the whistle on our appetite for delicious foods when they seem inappropriate.

It hasn't yet, so let's continue the meal with appetite, relish the flavours in the daal, the textured sweet, tart and salty vegetables, the ineffable umami in the silky gravy of lentils. The luxurious creaminess of dahi is yet to come, but will there be room for it?

Appetite has been receding for a while now. We eat slowly, conversation picks up again. Seconds are reluctantly refused.

The actual volume of food I've eaten is small, nowhere near the capacity of my stomach, but I'm beginning to feel full. I think I'll pass on that last shred of roti, and no dahi for me, thanks.

Why am I feeling full?

With the first morsel swallowed, my stomach has broadcast the news down the small intestine. The intestine responds with what can only be described as a chemical symphony, a cascade of chemicals all of which carry only one message: ENOUGH!

In protest, the stomach secretes the ONLY appetite-enhancing chemical in the gut—ghrelin.

Among the other sort are hormones from the pancreas, from the gall bladder, from the cells in the intestinal lining. As they're secreted into the bloodstream, they arrive in a heartbeat at the arcuate nucleus and convey their message.

Ghrelin also turns up to say its piece.

There is urgency in this argument of gut hormones sloshing against the arcuate nucleus. The decision is awaited: *Enough, or more?*

As if this cacophony weren't sufficient, nutrients from my meal—sugars, fats and amino acids—declare themselves too. The arcuate nucleus delivers its decision in a flush of hormones that reduce appetite. It is joined by the solitary tract nucleus in the midbrain to strengthen this signal, and I begin to feel full. I am satiated.

Satiation is the word used to describe the termination of eating a meal.

Satiety is a more long-term affair, and we know how that story goes, with leptin and insulin as its principal players.

We linger, chatting lazily, and then somebody remembers—dessert's waiting in the fridge.

We couldn't possibly, not now.

What *is* it?

Oh?

Oh!

Well, just a little, I guess.

Somebody checks on the dessert and returns to say, it hasn't set yet, give it half an hour more.

We clear the table, do the dishes, and return to conversation.

None of us really wants dessert, but I'm surprised how often we allude to it in a conversation that has nothing to do with food.

At some point, all pretense pretence vanishes and the talk becomes entirely about dessert.

A soft melancholy suffuses the air. There's music faraway. Long digested desserts are resurrected in memories that aren't about food. Forgotten neighbours and ghostly relations make guest appearances. Then someone notices the moon at the window and we smell the first stars of jasmine on the vine.

At this point, in the hush that equally unites and separates us, the dessert is brought in.

Orexis* was a Greek god who ate himself sick—

No, he wasn't.

---

*No, it isn't the herbal male enhancement pill—the wishful admixture of catuaba bark, ginseng, yohimbe, horny goat weed and tribulus—that promises strength and hardness in an erection. When will man learn that the largest sex organ is the brain?

We have the rights on that one. Kumbhakarna, remember him? (The *Ramayana* is an ever-reliable desk reference on obesity.)

Kumbhakarna was a good-hearted demon who ate like a pig, hibernated for months, and woke up in a confused rage. A hypothalamic disorder there, most definitely.

Medical textbooks eagerly scan the world's memory for diseases, but they have missed out on Kumbhakarna. We read instead of the fat boy Joe in Dickens' *Pickwick Papers*, described in perfectly observed clinical detail.

No, Orexis was not a greedy Greek.

We're all familiar with Anorexia Nervosa, as a disease. Anorexia simply means a lack of appetite.

In common parlance we seldom use the back-formation, *orexia* as an opposite. Bulimia is the commoner word.

Orexin is a neat term for the appetite-inducing chemicals secreted by the hypothalamus.

The other sort are Anorexins.

This is the chemical response to the metabolic drive. Half an hour ago, the verdict was anorexia. We were satiated by a good meal. We had explicit orders to stop eating. But the hypothalamus had reckoned without dessert.

The dessert is pretty. It has a luscious topping of fruit. There is a golden glint of caramel. Within its shiny kamarbandh of chocolate, a creamy mound wobbles delicately.

It knocks loudly on that other pathway in my brain, the reward circuit.

The sated hunger circuit is now at odds with the excited reward wiring.

As a high-sugar-high-fat food, the dessert has every evolutionary blessing that should convince the hypothalamus, if pleasure is insufficient argument.

The conversation between 'hunger' and 'pleasure' ends with 'like' becoming 'want'.

The attractions of the dessert have overridden the STOP signal from the rest of the body. The hypothalamus switches on its orexins once again, and I enjoy dessert.

The flurry of delighted compliments has given way to a meditative silence.

A creamy cloudlet trembles on each raised spoon. We're all eating the same dessert, but each of us is tasting something different.

I'm tasting the only dessert I know.

I'm seven years old.

It is very dark outside, not yet 5 a.m. It is the first day of Ramadan and my first roza.

I'm bursting with excitement, hunger is the last thing on my mind.

My mother is busy in the kitchen. She catches sight of me, hands me a bowl and goes back to the stove.

I take it wordlessly. The quickest way to freedom is to eat without questions.

With the first spoonful, the world stops.

Nothing exists but the heaven in my mouth.

It has no other name.

It is a rain-drenched cloud, a flower unfurling on my tongue, a scoop of moon in my spoon. Soft, creamy, sweet, gone.

My mother doesn't say a word. I don't either.

It is our secret, nobody else has ever tasted it, nobody else ever will.

Every morning through that month, that bowl delivered its magic.

We never talked about it.

I never did ask my mother what it was. I didn't need to. I knew right then, on that first Ramadan morning, that it was the most delicious food in the world.

It still is.

I crave it every time I eat dessert, and sometimes, like tonight, I taste its simplicity and its depth again.

Like the others, I'm eating this dessert not only because it is delicious, but because my brain unlocks a past deliciousness that I cherish. I'm not eating sugar and cream, but the memory of an experience of sugar and cream.

Foods which are perceived as intensely pleasurable are super-stimuli that scoff at free will. They ignore satiety signals. We just go ahead and eat them.

How much is the question—how much is *enough*?

Very few obese people consider themselves large eaters. Most aren't, and are deeply saddened by friendly advice to 'eat less'.

And yet, obesity begins with dietary excess.

Yes, it is compounded by insulin resistance which prevents energy utilization, but one cannot ignore that build-up of dietary excess.

Many people over-eat under stress. There is a ready explanation for this. In conditions of stress, a hormone in the brain (Corticotrophin Releasing Factor, CRF) drives an appetite for palatable foods. These are, inevitably, high-energy foods.

So, over-eating is specifically limited to foods that will build up an 'energy excess'.

CRF also drives a compulsion to eat when we see alluring images of food. The vast popularity of cooking shows provides endless visual incentive.

The same pattern operates in 'joyous eating' too. Good news, reunions, deeply satisfying emotions, these can all trigger CRF and impel us to search for a treat. And what do we celebrate with but something rich, creamy, sweet and—rewarding!

There is some, but not enough, evidence to show that in obese people the levels of pleasure are not achieved quickly;

this makes them overeat, and overeat in particular, high-energy foods packed with fat and sugar.

'But I hate sweets!' is a familiar protest, and not without reason. Why then pile on kilos? The answer, of course, is in the fat that makes salty snacks so delightful.

There is also evidence that the satiety signals from the gut are ignored by the hypothalamus in the obese. This could mean that an obese person relies solely on gastric distention to cease eating, and continues to eat till his stomach is full. '*Pet bhar gaya*' in such cases, is a literal truth.

It seems likely that the same set of signals operate in obese and non-obese people to terminate a meal, but obese people respond differently.

So do the non-obese, when faced with high-energy foods saturated with fats and sugar.

Look around—almost every food in sight is survival food, the kind we hope to have on us when we are stranded in the Himalaya or cast adrift at sea.

And here struts in the problem—when pleasure is blunted, one eats more.

One eats more of what is pleasurable.

To me, the most striking feature of Metabolic Syndrome is not obesity, but anhedonia, the lack of delight. It shows through the chinks in that armour of good humour, friendliness and warmth. It is struggling to express itself, and is invariably mistaken for unhappiness—which of course it also is.

But anhedonia is much more unbearable than unhappiness. It is the loss of sentience and perception.

We walk past unmoved by a child's laugh, a flower, a distant birdcall.

Life loses its uncertainties, its madcap frivolities, and assumes a rigid grey grid.

Joy leaches out of us. Listlessly, we nibble a bar of chocolate, and before we know it, it's gone.

The Taste of Fat

Do we actually taste *fat*, in the manner we taste sweet, salt, bitter, tart and umami?

Sweet as in sugar, salt as in table salt, bitter as in karela, umami as in meat—fat as in *what?*

What does the tongue perceive in that delicious bite of a flaky samosa?

A good samosa is all about its spicy contents. But the samosa nonpareil is all about *promise*. It is about how the samosa sits, elegant and equilateral, its lapel zipped. The central bulge is evident, but ignorable. The crust is everything.

Pick it up, and the fingertips register the faintest give on gentle pressure: crisp, not soggy.

Its warm exhalation says toasty, sweet.

You know what it is going to taste like even before it touches your lips.

At first nibble, crunchy.

It spatters in melting flakes on the tongue.

Now what?

Salt?

Sweet?

Or simply *fat*?

This is the samosa nonpareil, remember, deep-fried to perfection. There is no question of your tongue meeting a greasy coating of thickened oil.

As the crust dissolves on the tongue, we are so ready for the next bite, we actually have to will ourselves to wait till we've swallowed. Everything in us declares, *How good that is!*

At this point, we haven't yet sorted out flavour, texture, taste. It just is *good*.

This unconditional approval taps into the evolutionary discrimination between *safe* and *unsafe*.

But to most of us, taste seems to have nothing to do about safety. It is all about pleasure.

And somewhere along the line, we've conditioned ourselves into thinking of taste as self-indulgent and hedonistic. The pleasure is much deeper because it is vaguely forbidden. While this becomes a deliciously guilty secret, the converse has become a loudly voiced belief: *Good food is not tasty.*

Why not listen to the body instead?

How good that is!

In evolutionary terms, Good = Safe = Tasty.

I think this simple equation has been subverted very recently, and that has a great deal to do with Indian obesity.

Traditionally, the simplest Indian meal relies very heavily on taste. A bowl of rice kanji or porridge is eaten with a piquant bite of pickle or a lick of chutney. Dry roti finds itself a bit of onion and green chilli. Upscale this, and we stumble into the inexhaustible larder of masalas, pickles, papads, chutneys, preserves, and things without name, without origin, which capture every nuance of odour and taste.

Taste Is Us.

Fat, as the fuel needed to grow a brain, was definitely wanted by the body. To put it another way, throughout evolution, the body craved fat.

How did the body recognize fat?

To return to the samosa nonpareil, take it for granted that the body's hearty approval was a response to the fat in it.

To make the perfect crust, the best samosa professional I know uses a fatty dough: one part of fat to five parts of flour. And the fat he prefers is vanaspati, hydrogenated vegetable oil, that works wonders for short crust. At 5 p.m., when he sets up his kadhai, he pours in a golden stream of refined oil, cranks up his pressure stove to an intense blue flame, and while the oil heats up, gets busy shaping the samosas. The rested dough is soft and pliant and his portions of filling opulent. Twelve plump samosas slide into the oil which erupts in a slurry of fine golden bubbles, like a Klimt painting.

Frying samosas is not the slapdash anyhow some people use for bhajiyas, he tells me, with the slightest emphasis on *some*. Samosas require patience.

While we're being patient, the kadhai has attracted passersby. Some stare, others quickly walk past. A few, like me, decide to wait.

When I finally receive the samosa nonpareil, still palpitant and exhaling steam, its aroma has me cringing with appetite.

And yes, it is perfectly fried, making its newspaper plate only slightly translucent.

When it crumbles in a flurry of flakes, my tongue instantly tastes the stuff that evolution has graded A—fatty acids in the crust. But vanaspati (and other cooking oils) don't contain free fatty acids. The fat in them is in the same form as in adipose tissue: Triacylglycerol (TAG).

So is it TAG that I taste? When I say *taste*, I don't mean the smell or feel of fat.

We taste salt, sugar and tart, bitter and umami, because we have cells with receptors that pick up these tastes, and translate them into electrical signals to the brain. These receptors are housed in papillæ—taste buds. There are thousands of them, not only on the tongue, but scattered all over the mouth—insides of the cheeks, palate, back of the throat.

Besides these basic sensations, the irritative tastes are recognized by a number of receptors—pepper/chilli, garlic, mustard all link up with different receptors. So, is there a receptor for fat?

Different fats have distinctive flavours, by aroma. But we can taste fat in only one form—free fatty acids. Even minuscule amounts of free fatty acids are perceived as a 'taste'.

Why would we need to taste fat?

Is there a feel-good factor in free fatty acid?Remember, also, this has nothing to do with nutrition. It is all happening in the mouth.

The feel-good factor is a chemical, a bliss molecule, similar to the pleasure chemicals in hashish (cannabis). Since these are produced inside the body, they are called endo-cannabinoids. One of them is tellingly named *anandamide*.*

Endo-cannabinoids are signalling molecules present in many body tissues, including the mouth. They enhance the perception of taste, and induce the brain to signal appetite.

They compel us towards the source of pleasure.

Endo-cannabinoids have a lot to do with the pleasure of eating sweets. Could they also give us a sense of delight in tasting fat?

I want to focus on one particularly Indian perception of dietary fat.

Until very recently, when a glut of Western desserts captured our appetite, the national preference for fat texture was *crisp*.

*Anandamide, N-arachidonoylethanolamine or AEA, is a fatty acid neurotransmitter derived from the non-oxidative metabolism of arachidonic acid. The name derives from the Sanskrit *ananda*, which means bliss or joy. The Czech chemist Lumír Ondřej Hanuš and the American pharmacologist William Anthony Devane first isolated and described it in 1992 while working at the Hebrew University of Jerusalem.

Our traditional cooking oils are prized for flavour. Regional cuisines rely on mustard (north and east), coconut (west), and sesame (south). These oils temper most dishes with a rich vein of flavour.

Dairy fat, butter, and ghee, are for luxury.

Yes, we are a ghee-soaked culture, but that is mostly aroma and pampering.

In contrast, the Western palate prizes fatty emulsions.

I make this point to focus on the impossibility, and unreliability, of generalization when it comes to taste perception.

Endo-cannabinoids or not, fat is pleasurable. In combination with sugar, even more so.

Children who will hesitate over unfamiliar foods are most receptive to sweets high in sugar and fat. A child who shudders at an egg will happily gorge on cake. A plain cake is not as attractive as an iced one even when it is very sweet, and a frosted cake is never quite as seductive as a cream pastry.

Cakes, in India, till about twenty years ago, were birthday events. Christmas and Easter brought darkly delectable fruit cakes, but it took a birthday for a chocolate cake bouffant with cream.

Birthdays were annual events—now there's a birthday every week at office, and, of course, it comes with cake.

On my street—which is far removed from the hub—there are four shops entirely dedicated to extravagant patisserie. Downhill, where the college crowd hangs out, every second shopfront flaunts an overdressed cake, and coffee shops offer gargantuan wedges of gateaux, and there are small kiosks that 'take orders' for cakes in haute couture. Many flaunt a boastful placard as anticipatory bail: NO eggs. 100 per cent vegetarian.

That is a lot of cake.

The standard recipe for a plain homemade cake is 1 cup of flour, 1 cup of sugar, half a cup of fat, one egg. You can fool around with the type of fat—butter, ghee, oil, eggs, cream, dahi. You can raise raise the fat for a more tender and lighter texture—but skimp on it and you'll end up with a brick. 'Vegetarian' cakes simply avoid eggs, up the oil, and pile on cream and dahi. And that's still very plain cake.

Soft icing is hydrogenated fat or butter and sugar.

Most birthday cakes have geological layers of 'cream,' each stratum an inch thick.

A half-kg cream cake takes the same weight of fat for the icing alone. That is an incredible 4,500 calories, *two days' requirement of energy in the icing alone.*

That doesn't really bother me. I'm only going to have a *piece* of cake.

A wobbly cream cake won't cut into slices unless it is frozen, but it cuts comfortably into wedges. Generous wedges. They'll buckle and collapse if too small.

I could still land up eating my energy requirement for the entire day in that piece of cake.

Just across from one of these patisseries on my road, Ram Kumar Yadav is setting up his jalebi stall. He looks barely sixteen, but his wrist work is enviable. The kadhai holds up to two litres of oil. Jalebis come up golden and crisp, with only the faintest sheen—perfectly fried.

'You can't use over-heated thickened oil for frying sweets,' he tells me. He passes it on to the samosa guy down the road, they have an arrangement.

The jalebis are plunged immediately into simmering syrup, and here they are, a mound of molten gold, crisp, juicy to the core, simply delectable.

And yet I've seen a respectable pastry chef shudder at a jalebi: 'Indian sweets? No thanks, too much sugar and fat. No imagination.'

I rest my case.

The Western palate, as I mentioned earlier, reads the acceptable mouthfeel of fat as a creamy emulsion, whether savoury or sweet. Don't just think butter icing. Think mayonnaise, think hollandaise sauce, think even a basic béchamel. Accordingly, most attempts to rectify foods overloaded with fat involve using additives that achieve the same mouthfeel of creaminess.

Our thinking brain, the orbito-temporal cortex, our most intellectual approach to fat, cannot discern between different fats, but is very discerning about texture. It can tell slither from grease. So a rat—or a human—fed an emulsion of castor oil, suitably flavoured, can mistake it for mayonnaise. I could even use a non-edible oil, and die convinced I overdosed on mayonnaise.

There's an entire industry devoted to exploiting this cerebral naïveté.

An important segment of food chemistry is devoted to the invention of fat substitutes. The purpose? To fool the brain into believing that you're eating fat when you're actually swallowing something *that only feels like fat.*

Fat substitutes are sneaked into commercial food products to provide the mouthfeel of fat without its bloated calorific value.*

These fat foolers can be gummy—carrageenen from seaweed, guar gum from cluster beans (gawar). They can be modified proteins made from eggs, whey, milk, gelatin. They can be carbohydrate based—maltodextrin, inulin, or from grain-based fibre.

These substitutes have their own energy values too, besides trailing a slew of other disadvantages.

'Fat free' and 'zero cholesterol' labelled foods may contain one or many of the above. Soups, spreads, sauces, yoghurts, ice-creams, fillings, all the endless array of 'healthy' foods

*9 calories/gm

on supermarket shelves, contain these fat substitutes in an attempt to indulge 'the human preference for fat'.

There are also fat-based substitutes for fats. No, that wasn't a typo.

These are large molecule fats—which cannot be absorbed by the intestine. So though they look, smell, taste and feel like the genuine article, they don't function like fats because they're on a bullet train from mouth to anus. They are widely used in the food industry—Olestra is commonly known. It is banned in many countries, because of discomfiting side-effects and a real danger of vitamin deficiency as fat-soluble vitamins A, D and K in foods cooked in this medium do not get absorbed.

The brain does bank on fat for pleasure. It prefers even more a meld of fat and sugar.

When did this begin?

I can imagine early *Homo* feasting on a fatty haunch of boar, but not baking a cake. That happened when we turned agrarian 10,000 years ago when butter became a premium food. In India, the ritualistic use of ghee and the charming myths of Krishna probably mark the place where fat became recognized for its delights. By 1500 B.C., Sushruta was recommending ghee for impending blindness, impotence and failing wits, besides sloshing it on almost everything the local pharmacy purveyed. Almost in the same breath, he cautioned against using too much, lest it lead to that dread disaster, obesity.

Our primitive urge for fat is only one of many primitive urges.

How many of these do we indulge without consequence? They have all been urbanized out of recognition. When they do erupt, it is unacceptable.

The human brain has failed to show any evolutionary progress in the last thousand years. Of course, it is too early to tell, but from the state of our planet it doesn't look as if our species is building a bigger or better brain.

Traditional cuisines were developed in accordance with climate, vegetation, and livestock. They were just perfect for the energy demands of place, time, and lifestyle. How many of us live in the same place where our great-grandparents did? Does our lifestyle approximate theirs?

Food, like everything else, needs to be customized to our lives, to our lifetimes. Chewing the fat is so yesterday.

Dietary Fats

What do we talk about when we talk about 'dietary fats.'?

Let's start in the kitchen.

Cooking oil. Is it liquid at room temperature? If it is, it is *unsaturated* fat.

Saturated fats are solid at room temperature.

Coconut oil is solid at room temperature, and so is vanaspati, hydrogenated fat.

Ghee is saturated fat. So is butter. Cheese has up to 50 per cent fat, so let's count it as such.

Nuts contain between 40 and 58 per cent fat.

Oil seeds, the usual seeds we use for tempering—mustard, methi, til—are all oil sources.

The *un*usual seeds, being promoted as 'health giving'—flax, chia, sunflower—have oil too.

In addition, milk and dahi/curds have fat—to find out how much, look at the percentage figure on the packet:

- Cow's milk, or standard toned 3 per cent milk, has 3 gm of fat for every 100 ml.
- Buffalo milk, or full cream milk, has anything between 6–8 per cent fat/100ml.

So a standard 200 ml glass of milk already contains 1 tsp of butter if it is toned milk, and almost 2 tsp if it is full-cream.

That's just the raw food. I'm leaving out the processed, the bottled, the tinned, and above all, the baked and the fried out of this equation.

With so many sources of fat, how does one decide what's good and what's not?

Switch on the TV, and the first commercial you're likely to see is one about a 'healthy' oil. There are oils marketed as 'heart healthy,' as diabetes preventives, as 'light,' as low-absorptive, and of course as 'zero cholesterol,' omega-rich and bursting with anti-oxidants. To help us navigate through this worrying terminology comes the devoted young wife who pledges her husband's health with a 15-litre keg of the perfect oil. It has every one of those mysterious ingredients and all you have to remember is the brand name. And in case you're not among the samosa-eating, murukku-munching hoi polloi, there is Mediterranean allure in that clear stream of olive oil being poured out on squirming pasta by the extra virgin posed alongside.

Begin with the commonest stuff, 'refined' oil.

The refinement is in the industrial treatment that leaves the oil clear, colourless, odourless, and with an extended shelf-life. The oil may be derived from groundnuts, safflower or sunflower, these being the commonest in India.

We think of all liquid oils as unsaturated fats, but they contain a little saturated fat too. They also contain varying amount of trans fats.

Linoleic acid (LA) and Alphalinolenic acid (ALA) are *essential* fats. They *must* be present in the diet as they cannot be manufactured in the body. They are metabolized into long-chain fats, arachidonic acid, eicosapentaenoic acid and docosahexaenoic acid, all of which have important functions in the body.

Mostly, animal fats are saturated. Vegetable fats, are unsaturated.

The cholesterol scare begun began with an epidemiological paper, the Seven Countries Study. Starting in 1958, cohorts from Finland, Netherlands, Croatia, Serbia, Greece, United States of America and Japan were examined for possible contributory factors to cardiovascular disease. This study linked a high serum cholesterol, obesity, hypertension and smoking to an increased incidence of heart attacks and strokes.

After dietary recommendations in the USA, fat content in the average American diet dropped from over 40 per cent in the 1970s to 34 per cent in the 1990s.

Meanwhile, Americans were eating much more of everything else, especially sugar. With the result that obesity and Metabolic Syndrome boomed. The facile conclusion drawn was that a reduction in dietary fat had only made things worse.

Americans had also been recommended to switch from saturated fats to unsaturated fats—from Crisco and butter to PUFA (Poly Unsaturated Fatty Acid) rich oils. An interesting method of tracing this is to read the change in standard recipes in American cookbooks.

Has it helped at all?

In essence, the diet-heart hypothesis states that reducing saturated fats in the diet and replacing them with oils rich in linoleic acid, reduces the risk of cardiovascular disease.

A review, fifty years later, questions this.

Yes, the serum cholesterol did fall significantly when saturated fats were replaced by oil rich in linoleic acid. But, shockingly, the mortality from cardiovascular illnesses actually went up.

That was the news from America.

In India, concurrently, the winds of change were felt too. From 1980 onwards, the shift away from traditional oils to refined oils took off. New products appeared on the market, and discouraged the use of saturated fats. Hydrogenated vegetable fats (Dalda was the pioneer) have been in the Indian market since 1937.

Vanaspati ghee is often shortened to just ghee in popular perception, especially in the north, where desi ghee specifies the genuine dairy article. Now refined oil, with a high PUFA content was all set to edge it out.

What is PUFA, polyunsaturated fatty acid, all about?

It is something we need to swallow.

MUFA, monounsaturated fatty acids and SFA, short chain or saturated fatty acids can be manufactured in the body, but not PUFA.

PUFA is an umbrella label: polyunsaturated fatty acids are long chain fatty acids.

It is worthwhile understanding how we arrive at their common names.

Many fatty acids have eighteen carbon atoms, and the double bonds are designated by position. Linoleic acid has eighteen carbon atoms and two double bonds, the last being six carbon atoms away from the methyl end of the molecule. This gives it a jawbreaker label we can ignore,* but also a smaller tag we must take note of. That small number relates to the last double bond. It is six carbon atoms away from the methyl end, so linoleic acid is an Omega-6 fat.

Alphalinolenic acid, ALA, another constituent of PUFA has its last double bond at position three, and so it is an Omega-3 fat.

Other Omega-3 fats are EPA (Eicosapentaenoic Acid) and DHA (Docosahexaenoic Acid).

Within the body, Omega-6 and Omega-3 compete for the same enzyme. If the PUFA in the diet contains too much of Omega-6, Omega-3 doesn't stand a chance. And both Omega-6 and Omega-3 can inhibit the processing of saturated fats.

Why do we need Omega-6 or Omega-3?

Omega-6 turns into arachidonic acid which goes on to make phospholipids essential to all cell membranes. The pathway for Omega-3 competes with this.

Omega-3 DHA is present in the brain and nervous tissue,

---

*(9Z,12Z)-octadeca-9,12-dienoic acid.

and it is vital to vision. It is also the stuff that builds the brain. Pregnant mothers must be ensured enough Omega-3 in their diet.

How do Omega-3 and Omega-6 achieve such complicated targets?

They form a group of chemicals called eicosanoids.* These twenty-carbon compounds make up a very focussed, rapid-action, vigilante group. Among the tricks they pull off are chemicals that tweak inflammation and immunity. This function is of great import in the development of obesity and Metabolic Syndrome, which, as we've seen, is a state of general inflammation. Needless to say, eicosanoids are seldom amicable with each other.

Eicosanoids derived from Omega-6 cause thrombosis and inflammation to a greater degree, compared to those derived from Omega-3.

Omega 6 increases WAT, and prevents the 'browning' of adipocytes. The biochemical fallout is predictable: insulin resistance, leptin resistance, reduced adiponectin secretion, raised triglycerides, Metabolic Syndrome—OBESITY?

Omega-3 does just the opposite. The good guys DHA and EPA encourage 'browning', reduce insulin resistance, and triglycerides.

Omega-6 encourages the liver to store fat.

Omega-3 stops the deposition of fat in muscles and, by increasing insulin sensitivity, allows them to efficiently utilize glucose for energy.

Remember those ananda-making chemicals, cannabinoids? Omega-6 messes them up, skews the pleasure factor, and makes us eat more. Omega-3, meanwhile, true to type, tries to mop up the damage.

Of course, besides all this important stuff, the fatty acids in PUFA also are burned up for energy.

---

* *Eicosa-*, Greek for twenty.

This takes place in the mitochondria of all cells (except the brain and kidneys).

PUFA needs more steps than saturated fatty acids to enter this energy cycle. A high-fat diet alters this energy cycle as well.

Here are some figures from the FAO (2015):

- In 1990, India had nearly 200 million malnourished people.
- In 2012/14 the figure has remained the same.

That is more than 35 per cent Indians in chronic energy deficit in a country that has 20 per cent in chronic energy excess.

In the early 1990s, the world figure for fat consumption/capita/day was 68.3 gm. Americans ate 151 gm/day.

In 2016, in India, rural Indians consume 19 per cent of their daily energy as fat, and urban Indians 26 per cent among women and 24 per cent among men.

Since the recommended amount is 15–30 per cent, it doesn't seem as though we're doing so badly. *This underlines how misleading statistics can be.*

Are we getting enough Omega-3?

The recommended amount is 200 mg/day.

Urban Indian women manage about 20 mg/day, and there's no telling about the rest of us.

In contrast, we seem to be taking in more Omega-6 than we really need to.

Return to our cheery TV housewife and look closer at the 15-kg can of oil she's cuddling. Safflower, sunflower, and groundnut are the commonest oils in use. Safflower and sunflower oil contain mainly Omega-6.

Researchers have raised this very obvious anxiety—Is the increasing consumption of Omega-6-rich oils responsible for the low levels of Omega-3 in all of us?

Groundnut oil, in common with olive oil, has oleic acid, Omega-9 stuff. Safflower and sunflower oils with high oleic acid are also on the market.

India's traditional oils are groundnut, sesame, mustard and coconut.

India is among the world's leading producers of rapeseed, a variant in the mustard family, and currently the most consumed oilseed on the planet. Both mustard and rapeseed oils have Omega-3, but also contain 20–50 per cent erucic acid which is toxic.

Oil from rapeseed, low in erucic acid and rich in Omega-3, is in our markets, and India produced 2.11 million metric tonnes in 2015–16, but we don't eat much of it.

Mustard oil, of the traditional sort, is the highest consumed oil in the country even though its use is restricted to the north and the east. It seems unlikely that other parts of the country will find rapeseed oil palatable—unless of course it is marketed as Canola, which being American, will be swallowed thirstily without question.

The other oil which has a strong Omega-3 presence is soya-bean oil. We imported 3.5 million tonnes of it in 2015–16, and presumably, ate it too. It is difficult to gauge its place in Indian cuisine. Deodorized out of all recognition, any edible oil can work. The news from research on soya oil is far from comforting. It is, definitely, obesogenic in rats—a reliable animal model for human obesity.

We imported 9.54 million tonnes of palm oil in 2015–16. Not a traditional oil, palm oil was introduced into our public distribution system several decades ago. Palm oil is high in saturated fats (51.5 per cent).

Coconut oil needs special consideration, but the others all contain a mixture of MUFA and PUFA.

Coconut oil is the cooking medium of choice in the Indian southwest, Kerala in the main.

In comparison with other cooking oils, it has some

important differences. It is solid at cool temperatures, indicating a high saturated fat content. Coconut oil is 91 per cent saturated fat, the highest in all cooking oils. It contains a special sort of fat—Medium Chain Triglyceride. MCTs don't require bile for their digestion. They are passively absorbed from the intestine and transported straight to the liver. This makes them a rich source of nutrition in the presence of intestinal disease.

Coconut oil is being promoted as a wonder food for the aging brain, and as a cardio-protective, despite its high saturated fat content.

It is noteworthy that Kerala, which fuels on coconut oil, has a high incidence of cardiovascular illness, diabetes and obesity, perhaps the highest in our country.

What is the optimum ratio of Omega-6 to Omega-3 in daily dietary fat intake?

Presently, the Indian consumption is 15:1.

A much lower ratio is recommended.

Lowering the ratio to 4:1, for instance, reduces cardiovascular risk.

Low ratios have also been linked with reduction in arthritis, asthma and—most significantly—breast cancer.

Just to check what this skewed ratio means in evolutionary terms, what were we eating 1.8 million years ago?

Surprise, surprise—fruit, nuts and berries all contained a serious amount of Omega-3 in those happy days. You could get your fix of DHA and EPA on your morning walk even if the day's hunting and fishing cheated you of prey.

The Omega-6: Omega-3 ratio in *Homo ergaster*'s lunch was 0.79:1.

It is surmised that till 200 years ago, when life became aggressively industrialized, we sustained ourselves by getting just 20 per cent of daily energy from fat. Now we average 40 per cent.

Saturated fat intake has increased. We are consuming more Omega-6 and less Omega-3.

For certain, this parallels the global rise in obesity.

There is incontrovertible evidence that increased Omega-6 intake triggers a pro-inflammatory state in the body, and it influences the adipocyte to tip all its resources in favour of obesity.

It also dampens the appetite regulatory effects of Omega-3.

Omega-6 increases endocannabinoids, and promotes the 'fatty high' that drives us to eat more, and eat more of fat and sugar.

Is this sufficient to criminalize Omega-6 as the reason for the obesity pandemic?

There is a lot more evidence to consider, especially evidence from our kitchens.

The fat most beloved by the human race is, undoubtedly, butter.

Butterfat is consumed joyously in India as milk, curds, lassi, cottage cheese (paneer), and, above all, as ghee.

Cheese is an acquired taste, but a rapacious one.

Then, there is khoya, evaporated milk, the very soul of our inexhaustible treasury of sweets.

Dairy is often the only source of protein in vegetarian households. At Rs 45+/litre in most cities, it is far from affordable for low-income households. The worst hit are children.

A glass of milk (200 ml) a day guarantees 6 gm of protein and 6 gm of fat, a small fraction of what a six-year-old needs, but most little ones don't get even that.

Our annual consumption of milk is 59.57 million metric tonnes.

How much of this is consumed as milk?

Only 46 per cent.

Ghee makes up 27.7 per cent.

Butter 6.5 per cent.
Curds 7 per cent.
The remainder 10 per cent are commercial products.

Dairy is saturated fat, and should, by all accounts, encourage atherosclerosis, diabetes and yes, obesity.

Recent studies question this wisdom.

Butter intake of between a teaspoon and a tablespoon a day didn't seem to raise the risk for heart disease and actually lowered the incidence of Type 2 diabetes. But the study also points out an important difference: evaluating foods can produce very different results from evaluating food components individually. While the effects of saturated fat are undeniable, butter as a food may offer benefits through compounds that counteract this. No matter how you dress that up, it is just a guess.

Dairy fat contains a small amount of a type of fat that is dangerous—trans fats.

Vanaspati/margarine, made by partially hydrogenating vegetable oils, can contain a staggering amount of trans fats.

Polyunsaturated fatty acids change their double bond configurations from *cis* to *trans* by partial hydrogenation.

Trans fats are, very nearly, saturated fats, and therefore solid at room temperature. Their higher melting point makes them ideal for frying and baking. This has been commercially exploited since 1911 when Crisco revolutionized American cooking.

Vanaspati and margarine are used very frequently. The entire food industry runs on hydrogenated oils. Crisp, flaky, tender, soft, you-name-it, and it is vanaspati. The bakery business would buckle under without it, as would all the melt-in-the-mouth snacks that swear they're made in ghee.

Trans fats raise serum LDL cholesterol, lower HDL cholesterol and alter the total cholesterol/HDL ratio. They also raise serum triglyceride levels. They are bad news in every manner, and what's worse, they increase the risk of cardiovascular disease.

They achieve harm by encouraging immune cells to release inflammatory chemicals, and by directly damaging the lining of capillaries. They alter metabolic processes within liver cells.

In the body, HDL is converted to LDL and VLDL (very low density lipoproteins) by an enzyme; an increase in trans fats in the diet activates this enzyme. This, in part, explains the blood picture on a high trans-fat diet: high levels of LDL and VLDL, low levels of HDL.

Predictably, trans fats cause the adipocyte to suspend making more triglycerides to increase its stores. Instead, it starts leaking free fatty acids and sets off Metabolic Syndrome.

Very low levels of trans-fat in the diet (1–3 per cent of total energy intake) are enough to cause substantial increase in cardiovascular risk. That means 1/2 to 1 teaspoon of trans fats/day.

How much is that exactly, in terms of a vanaspati or margarine? Will a food label tell us?

Zero trans fats on the label means the product contains less than 500 mg of trans fats per serving. That is less than 1/10th of a teaspoon.

How much trans fats does a vanaspati or margarine contain?

It could be as high as 50 per cent of total fat!

As vanaspati is all fat, that is 1/2 teaspoonful (tsf) of trans fats in every spoonful!

Do I hear you protest?

You're right—most brands contain much less. In fact, Dalda, the pioneer brand of vanaspati, was also the first to earn itself a 'zero trans' label.

In 2009, the Food Safety and Standard Authority of India (FSSAI) proposed regulating the permissible levels of trans fats in vanaspati to 10 per cent and scaling it down further over the next few years. (Other countries have a ceiling of 2 per cent.)

With some oil companies responding to the challenge by reducing trans fats, FSSAI was able to further it by clamping the upper limit at 5 per cent in 2014. This has been in practice since 2016.

A community survey on trans fats and public awareness, conducted by the Indian Institute of Public Health, showed very clearly that household consumption of vanaspati in cooking was low, but the consumption of 'bought' snacks was high. And snacks of all varieties were high in trans fats. The study also brought out the importance of making small vendors and manufacturers of snack foods aware of the dangers of trans fats.

So is that it, then?

Is the world obese because we're eating the wrong sorts of fat?

But nobody really eats *just* fat—so there must be more to the story.

This, That, and the Other

The body has a shadow self.

Our shadow moves in us, with us, and, as is now becoming apparent, moves us. It could almost be a penumbra to free will.

It takes up its residence in the body even before we enter the world with our first cry of protest. It outlasts life. It is the body's only witness to the moment of death. It records that event in every corner and crevice of the body, and broadcasts the news so that a death, no matter how solitary, ignoble, or humble, can ever pass unnoticed.

From its emanations the footsteps of strangers stall in a moment of awed acknowledgment before they hurry past in terror, having sensed a mortality inseparable from their own.

The body's shadow writes the script for the dissolution after death.

What if it wrote the script for life itself?

It probably does.

This shadow is the universe that inhabits us. We are legion. We contain legions. Every part of our body exposed to the air is garrisoned, but the contingent I want to talk about is in our intestine. It occupies the lining of the small and large intestines.

Shadows are insubstantial.

In 1907, Duncan MacDougall of Haverhill, Massachusetts, conducted a bizarre experiment. He placed a dying man on a bed with a specially constructed weighing beam to measure the loss of weight immediately following death. He repeated this on five others and came up with a figure: 3/4^{ths} of an ounce—21 gm.

A similar experiment conducted on dogs revealed no loss of weight immediately after death.

On the Christian presumption that dogs have no souls, Dr MacDougall concluded: 'The net result of the experiments conducted on human beings, is that a loss of substance occurs at death not accounted for by known channels of loss. Is it the soul substance? It would seem to me to be so.'

Dr MacDougall has long been laughed out of medical history, but our shadow self is just beginning to make medical history. Unlike the soul, it has very real and very visible substance. It makes up 1–2 kg of body weight and consists of trillions of microorganisms cushioned on our intestinal cells and dipping their toes into intestinal contents. There are bacteria, viruses, protozoa, archaea and practically every form of unicellular life, in addition to more complex organisms like helminths, often rudely called worms.

Of all these, the most assertive seem to be the bacteria of two large phyla: *Bacteroidetes* and *Firmicutes*.

Together, the body's shadow population makes up the *microbiome*. It is as distinctive as a fingerprint, and we've only just begun to read the microbiome primer. While we discover, every day, a new way in which the microbiome runs our body, we know very little about how it pulls this off.

How does the microbiome control metabolism?

The crucial role it plays in human health was discovered, naturally, through mice. Mice are coprophagic—that's just politesse for 'they happily eat fæces'. Genetically germless mice, when they are fed on the excrement of obese mice, acquire that microbiome, and as a result, turn obese themselves.

This observation starts off a labyrinthine enquiry of *how*.

The microbiome is as individualistic as the genome, and

its effects on metabolism are variable. It is equally affected by environmental factors, and its immediate environment is its vast feeding pool. The intestine is a very long and a very lavish lunch, and the menu is what we have swallowed.

Earlier in this book, we saw how gut signals control satiation: they tell us when to stop eating. These signals emanate from intestinal cells in response to intestinal contents. The microbiome behaves in the same manner. Depending on what's for lunch, the microbiome secretes its own group of signalling molecules, many of which are fatty acids.

These act locally on intestinal cells, but much more curious are their distant effects—on the brain. These microbiome signals slip into the bloodstream, and arrive at those parts of the brain we're now familiar with—the nuclei in the hypothalamus. And there they tweak the secretion of orexins which make us eat and also the anorectic chemicals that make us desist from eating. The microbiome controls both appetite and satiation.

It has an equal, if not stronger, control over satiety—which determines when we next get hungry after a meal. This is accomplished by altering the leptin-ghrelin balance.

The microbiome of obese people shows distinctive differences from that of those with normal body weight.

The obese microbiome is deficient in bacteria from the phylum Bacteroidetes.

Bacteroidetes are specialists in breaking down complex plant sugars.

Firmicutes deal with simple sugars.

Obese microbiota extract more energy out of intestinal contents: they make possible the digestion of carbohydrates and proteins which would otherwise be extruded as indigestible. They alter bile acid metabolism, and this in turn raises insulin resistance and promotes high blood blood-sugar levels.

Obese microbiota also change the adipocyte, induce less fat storage, and thus free up more fatty acids into the circulation. They also alter the level of choline which is necessary for the synthesis of VLDL.

Intestinal bacteria liberate acetate, a short-chain fatty acid. Acetate acts on the brain to suppress appetite. In obese microbiota, the levels of acetate drop to cause just the opposite: over-eating and high sugar levels.

Obese microbiota can be reversed to normal flora by altering the diet to a medium- or low-energy one.

These facts make it evident that the microbiome is diet-dependent.

One more instance of proving that old adage: *your bacteria are what you eat*.

Polyphenols, present in nuts and fruit, accumulate in the large intestine and sustain a normal microbiome. High dietary protein, especially animal protein, eaten with very little fibre—the classic 'Western diet', shifts the normal microbiome into an obese profile.

In fact, the microbiome seems to shadow every change that leads up to Metabolic Syndrome.

Bacteria know every trick in the book, but do they cause obesity? Or does obesity cause an alteration in the microbiome?

This chicken or egg controversy hogs the discourse on obesity. Here too, a necessary caution. These observations, especially about the bacterial phyla reported, are from Western populations.

Various geographic regions have distinct human microbiota, and it is necessary for us to have a suitable Indian frame of reference. Much research is afoot, only a few results have been published. Healthy Indians have a rich abundance of the genus *Prevotella* that breaks down complex plant protein; *Lactobacillus*, a common fermenter; and *Megasphaera* which is common in ruminants.

Translated: We are vegetarian, we eat fermented foods, and we love milk.

Indians are, additionally, a more heterogeneous group with widely different diet preferences.

We have learnt the difference between white and brown adipose tissue—but these distinctions are at the microscopic level.

To the naked eye, adipose tissue looks radiantly yellow. It has the luxurious depth of egg yolk, every adipocyte a drop of sunshine.

I remember my first glimpse of living fat. How pretty it looked, as I peered over the shoulder of a senior surgeon. He clearly did not share my opinion as he charred his way past a thick wad of abdominal fat with an electrocautery. I have never heard a surgeon say, 'That's fat.' It is always, 'That's justfat.' In surgi-speak, justfat is one word.

If you're not a surgeon yourself, nor a chef, take my word for it. Fat *is* pretty. Think tiny egg yolks winking up at you, glistening, and gorgeously yellow.

Why *yellow*?

For that matter, why is egg yolk yellow?

The answer is on my window sill.

Huddled in the dappled shade of my pepper vine is a week-old pigeon fledgling. This morning she looks enormous compared to the pink-and-yellow weakling that peeped out from beneath her mother's wing last weekend. She's beginning to show grey coloration like her parents, though her baby down is still very visible. She's muscular, those pectorals are flashy already, and when she attempts to raise a shoulder, I catch a glimpse of her supracoracoideus muscle bulking up for flight. She staggers about the sill curiously while her parents look on with pride.

The crow that had exhibited a criminal interest in her last week, now keeps a respectful distance. She claims the world with a regal insouciance as she toddles in and out of the dangling vine. Princess Pepperina, ready for her fairy tale.

Compare her with a week-old human infant, completely helpless without adult care.

Princess Pepperina is a precocial fledgling—precocious in growth and development. And the reason for such precocity is the smart manner in which her mother nourished her.

A pigeon's egg is over 40 per cent yolk.

So, why is yolk so yellow?

Rapid growth causes a high amount of Reactive Oxygen Species (ROS) to accumulate. This endangers the embryo with oxidative stress which can destroy DNA, the proteins, and the lipids of developing tissue.

Carotenoids give the yellow colour to yolk, and they are strong anti-oxidants.

Bird eggs evolved anti-oxidant-enriched yolk to support the rapid growth of their embryos.

Yolk concentration of carotenoids varies with the rate of embryo growth, and so it is different in different species of birds.

Carotenoids also give human adipose tissue its yellow colour.

Why do we need so much of this stuff?

It is a question those of us who handle living tissue cannot evade.

It is also something that we need to know when we consider the changes of obesity.

What are carotenoids?

The yellow in carrots, certainly, but also the colouring in other bright yellow or red vegetables and fruit.

Our body does not manufacture carotenoids. They have to be eaten, and luckily for us, the plant kingdom is booming with them. Six hundred types and counting, forty of which are regular human fodder.

They have musical names—β-carotene, lycopene, β-carotene, β-cryptoxanthin, lutein, zeaxanthin, but there's little point in remembering them. Except the charm.

All carotenoids protect cells against oxidative damage. Many of them are precursors for Vitamin A, which behaves more like a hormone than a vitamin.

What does this have to do with adiposity?

A high-fat diet exposes the liver to a high fat load, and to fat deposition and fibrosis. As obesity sets in, this is compounded by the leak of fatty acids from overburdened adipocytes, and high levels of circulating triglycerides. The liver then begins to accumulate fat. With growing insulin resistance, the utilization of glucose, as well as oxidation of fats for energy is impaired.

High sugar levels, high insulin levels, and high triglyceride levels result in high VLDL and low HDL levels, a picture of complete dyslipidemia. Non Alcoholic Fatty Liver Disease (NAFLD) is the term for this complication of obesity. It is reversible. Liver cells are not, yet, irredeemably damaged.

Should the fatty liver cells swell up further and break, the liver will show signs of inflammation, and the stage is set for a far more serious condition, one which can lead on to fibrosis with the destruction of liver cells, resulting in cirrhosis and liver failure. This condition, Non Alcoholic Steato Hepatitis (NASH) is common in India, and like NAFLD, is strongly correlated with Metabolic Syndrome and obesity.

Carotenoids absorbed from the fruit and vegetables we eat are mainly stored in adipocytes. So adipose depots are storage sites for anti-oxidants that protect against oxidative stress. Carotenoids are particularly protective to the liver. And it's a fair guesstimate that Vitamin A metabolism is managed by the adipocyte.

It has been observed that obese adipocytes have lower levels of ß-carotene than healthy adipocytes. A similar low value has been observed in adipocytes from diabetic patients who are also obese. Yet, total body stores of ß-carotene are constant, irrespective of BMI.

There is growing evidence that the intake of Vitamin A is low in obese people.

Vitamin A deficiency is widespread in India, and so is obesity.

Coincidence?

Cause and effect?

Feeding obese rats with a diet rich in Vitamin A makes them lose weight.

This is just one more piece in the puzzle of obesity, but it might turn out to be an important one.

With such an overwhelming surge in obesity across the planet, is there a common factor in the environment acting as a driver for this emergence?

Fat has the unique property of dissolving many substances that are water-insoluble.

Such substances, when ingested, can be absorbed directly or after being dissolved in a dietary fat. Either way, they can enter the circulation of both blood and lymph and follow the same metabolic path as other ingested fats. Accordingly, they can be absorbed into the adipocyte and stored in its oil droplet.

Pesticides are everywhere. We have known of their lethal effects since the 1960s, when Rachel Carson published her observations in *Silent Spring*. Today we refer to them as Persistent Organic Pollutants or POP.

DDT spraying was banned in the US in 1972, but continues unabated in India.

DDT, and its metabolites, are found in above-permissible levels in the breast milk of Indian mothers.

POPs travel up the food chain. We eat them in fruits, vegetables, milk, meat and fish.

A global ban on DDT by the year 2020 was proposed in 2013. India vetoed it.

DDT spraying was the mainstay of our National Program for Malaria Control for five decades. It still continues, including indoor spraying (with the blessing of the WHO).

At the start of the twenty-first century, we were using 2,131,049 kg/year of DDT.

India is the only country still producing DDT. Even China stopped making it in 2007.

What is DDT, and why should it affect humans at all?

Dichlorodiphenyltrichloroethane, to use its formal name, is water insoluble, fat soluble and hangs around in the atmosphere for a very long time. Its metabolite, DDE, has a half-life of eleven years.

Imagine what it has done to birds by concentrating in egg yolks.

And what of us?

Fifty years of exposure should be enough to establish its link with disease, but considering various vested interests lobbying for the continued use of DDT, such links are, if not totally discredited, relegated to the back burner as 'possible, but unproven'.

We are willing to overlook the global increase in breast cancer, pancreatic and liver cancers, infertility in both sexes, complicated pregnancies, abortions, perinatal deaths, neuro-developmental delays in children, trans-generational breast cancers from *in utero* exposure to maternal DDT, congenital abnormalities of the genitals in boys, pre-senile dementias, and perhaps obesity too, for the questionable benefit of killing mosquitoes and agricultural pests.

The sentence that reappears with numbing regularity is, 'No adverse effects were reported in the exposed population.'

That should, more honestly, read, 'No adverse effects were *identified* in the exposed population.'

What should we be looking for?

DDT spray is wafted on air currents all the way up to the Arctic, so the effects are global, even if the use is only in the tropics.

It enters all aquatic forms of life and travels up the food chain, and concentrates in fish. The same is true of terrestrial life, and of course, birds.

DDT dissolves in fat, so it enters the fat metabolism of all these organisms, and the more fat there is, the greater the body store of ingested DDT.

The main metabolite of DDT, DDE, is a recognized 'hormone disrupter'. Its role as a blocker of androgen receptors is undisputed. It has been correlated with an increased incidence of hypospadias, low sperm counts, and testicular cancer. Even worse, DDE has been implicated in the births of babies with brain malformations and poor neurological development.

The breast is a very dynamic organ. Its cell composition and architecture change repeatedly throughout life. It has a very high concentration of adipose tissue, and POPs tend to get concentrated in breast tissue. After the age of forty, the glandular element of the breast wanes and is replaced by fat and fibrous tissue. In obesity, fat stores in the breast increase.

Breast tissue is under hormonal control, principally influenced by oestrogen. Any 'hormone disrupter' will disturb the regulation of adipocytes in the breast and prepare the stage for cancerous change. Both POPs and obesity can be linked with the rising incidence of breast cancer.

POPs are also implicated in the emergence of obesity. Their metabolites retard the maturation of adipocytes. When there is dietary excess, absorbed fat results in hypertrophy of adipocytes, early cell death, and leakage of fatty acids into the circulation.

POPs are concentrated in the oil droplet within the adipocyte—the more fat in there, the greater the amount of POP that can be held in solution. So obese individuals have large depots of entrapped POP. They may also have no detectable POPs in circulation as compared to lean people. This means that entrapped POPs in fat depots don't get to the more crucial organs in the body. The fat depots in obesity act as protective sinks for POPs.

One of the richest sources of POPs in the diet is fish. Fish high in fats like mackerel, hilsa, ghol and salmon can have alarmingly high levels.

Experimentally, a fish diet rich in POPs causes abdominal obesity and insulin resistance in rats within the fortnight.

Physiological reports bristle with instances of how POPs can disrupt adipocyte metabolism and cause Metabolic Syndrome—but no one is listening.

Now that other very real worry. What happens when we *lose* fat?

There is a real risk of the POPs sequestered in adipose depots breaking loose and entering the blood.

People who have lost weight abruptly and extremely—following liposuction or bariatric surgery—show high levels of circulating POPs and run the risk of organ damage.

Isn't there something *genetic* about obesity?

In a group of people of the same age and physical parameters, exposed to similar environments and eating the same food, why should only some turn obese? What sets them apart?

Surely it must be *genetic*.

I have italicized the word to emphasize how it has become a catch-all for everything metamagical and inexplicable. One can get out of almost any sticky situation by blaming it on genes.

What are the facts?

To date, more than forty genetic variants have been

associated with obesity and fat distribution. But these don't really explain the patterns of the heritability of obesity.

It is likely there are factors which influence the expression of genes without altering their DNA. Such factors are called *epigenetic marks*, as they act around a particular genetic profile. It is believed that environmental effects *in utero* cause epigenetic variations, which lead on to alterations in the metabolism.

Children of obese mothers are prone to obesity as they grow.

Weight reduction in obese women before pregnancy eliminates such an association.

It isn't yet clear what factors in obese mothers cause epigenetic change in the foetus.

If that sounds rather vague, that's because it *is* vague.

Clearly, this obesity pandemic is not a genetic disease, but neither is it free of genetic association.

It is not an environmental disease, but POPs are obesogenic.

We know that the gut microbiome is altered in obesity, but is it cause or effect?

It could all be this, that, and the other.

None of these possibilities interest me. They lack street cred.

I am not willing to ignore what is happening around me. Simple things. Things so obvious we ignore them as self-evident. Things that explain the epidemic of obesity, Metabolic Syndrome and diabetes.

Obesity, no matter what its cause, is about food.

So back to the kitchen we go.

Sugar, Sugar, Everywhere

India is the second-largest producer of sugar in the world, and we export a lot of it. We consume 18.9 kg/capita annually on an average. That works out to 50 gm/day—ten teaspoons.

We also glut on jaggery (gur) and candy (khandsar). As our consumption of gur and khandsar has dipped, our consumption of sweetened bottled drinks has zoomed. One can of a sweet aerated drink has as much as 35 gm of sugar.

India consumes an awful lot of sugar.

Yes, I know, others eat more. Brazilians the most, but our role model, the US of A, is way up there! And our, 'We're so much better than the West' attitude has earned us obesity and Metabolic Syndrome. 'Indian culture' is killing us in more ways than I can count, but I want to examine this in terms of sugar.

Again, I prefer the ground view. Statistics don't mean a damn thing. The only way out of this mess is a 'my life, my body' perspective.

Back to the kitchen, then.

To sugar, of course, and gur.

A bar of chocolate in the fridge.

Biscuits.

That's the usual list in 'health conscious' homes.

The sugar may not even be of the usual sort, but organic, non-bleached, brown, Demerara.

The jaggery may be palm sugar.

The biscuits may be cookies.

There is also tetra-pak juice, jam, sauces, cans of cola.

No?

Dried fruits, then?

Not common kishmish, raisins, but 'healthy stuff'. Apricots, sultanas, dates, prunes—with nuts alongside, without doubt.

A jar of honey—pure sunshine?

Malted powders, drinking chocolate?

Energy bars?

Syrups?

Spreads?

Condensed milk?

Chyawanprash?

Sugar, sugar, sugar—all sugar! For god's sake, gimme a life!

And, here's the rub. We have been looking at the kitchen on an ordinary day.

No guests. No festivals. No celebrations.

That's just at home.

What happens at the office? All those chais add up, cutting, masala, adrak, whatever, there is always sugar.

I'm at the school gate, watching the feeding frenzy.

At the exhilarating moment of liberation, the urgency is always for something sweet.

'Chinese bhel' has no aficionados at this hour. Locally made candy—shakkar para, laddu, chikki—has few takers unless it is sealed in plastic.

With the smaller children, buying power still lies in the hands of the mother, and she's a stickler for hygiene. She'll buy anything in a packet, even if it costs a rupee more.

Delectable rainbow candy, squishy bite-sized jujubes, chewy toffee, melting eclairs, bubble-gum, chewing gum—and we haven't even got to chocolate yet. Everything neatly sealed in colourful plastic or tinsel to delight the maternal heart. However much she might baulk at buying candy, very few mothers will hesitate over a packet of cream biscuits.

Older children? They have pocket money, and surprisingly, their choices aren't very different.

That *is* an awful amount of sugar.

What is it doing to us?

Cane sugar, those white granules in the kitchen tin, is sucrose, a disaccharide. It has two kinds of sugar. Glucose and fructose.

As the sweet I eat passes down my intestine, it meets up with the enzyme sucrase, which cracks sucrose into the two constituent sugars, glucose and fructose. Glucose, as we know, whistles up insulin once it enters the circulation. From then on, insulin regulates the entry of glucose into cells, to be used up for energy.

Fructose breaks free of insulin, and takes a direct hike to the liver. Here, it can be converted into compounds used for triglyceride and cholesterol synthesis. Very simply, fructose helps the liver make fat.

As fat synthesis increases, the levels of triglycerides in the blood rises.

Insulin resistance invariably accompanies high triglycerides, and, hey presto—Metabolic Syndrome!

Obviously, this doesn't happen with modest amounts of sugar in the diet.

How much is too much?

Most published studies have a snag. They ignore caloric excess from other sources and restrict observations only to 'free sugar' ingested. All caloric excess contributes to Metabolic Syndrome and its complications.

The conclusion from American studies is that the average American daily intake of sugar—15 per cent of daily energy consumed—raises cardiovascular risk by 18 per cent.

A very modest American daily intake would be 3,000 calories, so it works out to 450 calories from sugar = 22½ tsf a day.

That seems a ridiculous amount to an Indian whose daily intake is 2 tsp in tea or coffee. But count all the hidden sources, and I'm willing to bet it will touch 5 tsp, even without 'sweets.'

The bad news is that the fructose fraction of sugar has its way with the liver irrespective of the body's energy status, since it is outside insulin's control.

Another dismaying finding is that sugar increases hypothalamic orexins, which drive us into overeating. And, it is more than just the hedonic effect of sweet taste.

The fructose molecule is comparatively more hedonic than our humdrum glucose. It drives us into eating more sugar, and also, eating more of everything.

Once habituated to a high amount of sugar, the pleasure dims, driving one to excess.

Yes, sugar can be addictive.

We do know how enjoyable sugar is. Not only does a sweet delight, it also relaxes and comforts. Part of that reaction is chemical. Fructose begs adrenaline to ease off, and we feel less stressed. These are everyday observations, everyday comforts, and it is discomfiting now to read of them as crimes.

The verdict, then?

We are, certainly, eating an insane amount of sugar, and it is only reasonable to cut back.

Also, certainly, too much sugar can cause the more dangerous complications of Metabolic Syndrome: fat deposition in the liver and its consequences, dyslipidemia and subsequent atherosclerosis.

Is this particularly relevant to us in India?

Sadly, yes.

As we learnt earlier, we develop Metabolic Syndrome at a

lower BMI than Westerners do, and we are more susceptible to its complications in the liver and cardiovascular system.

Presently, Americans are being recommended a 'free sugar' cut off at 10 per cent of the day's energy consumption, and that is still 15 tsp/day.

Indian recommendations are lower—5 per cent of the day's energy consumption. That is still a large amount of 'free sugar'.

But, who's listening?

The European story of sugar is steeped in blood and tyranny, for it was sustained by the Slave Trade.

The Indian story of sugar has no such tragedies in its past, but its present is sustained by neocolonialism, and I am fearful about its future.

Nonetheless, I am as reluctant to criminalize sugar as I am to criminalize fat in our present pandemic of obesity.

The Quotidian

It is ironic the 2017 Nobel for Medicine and Physiology was awarded for a discovery which may well be tomorrow's answer to today's pandemic. Twenty-seven years ago, in 1990, Jeffrey Hall and Michael Rosbash of Brandeis University, and Michael Young of Rockefeller University, described a gene in the fruit fly that controls circadian rhythms—or as it is more snappily called—the body clock.

The body clock in the brain is a cluster of neurons, the suprachiasmatic nuclei, just above where the optic nerves cross. Think of it as an inch behind your eyes. Injure this area, and one can no longer tell night from day—not in terms of light perception, but in terms of sleep and wakefulness.

However, every individual neuron in this group is also an autonomous clock, set just a little out of sync with its neighbour.

That is an elegant, if surreal, concept.

I'm uncomfortable at the thought of a central all-seeing clock metering my every move. I find our present-day surveillance of spaces public and private morally abhorrent, deeply inimical to the sanctity of human liberty. A corrosion of trust runs in parallel with insularity and isolation, and leads inevitably to the fragmentation and collapse of societies. The last thing I could live with would be in-built surveillance, so I'm cheered by the thought that each one of my trillion or more cells has a clock of its own. The body micromanages life—or metabolism, if one insists on talking science.

The 'body clock' then refers to a collective regulator of all cell processes, harmonizing them with the sleep-wake cycle.

During sleep, insulin levels fall. Glucose is conserved for exclusive use by the brain. The rest of the body uses fat as fuel. When we wake, insulin levels rise. We eat. Dietary sugar powers our daily activities.

That is just the blueprint. How well do we keep to it?

The sleep-wake cycle is ordered by light. We are designed to wake with first light and sleep soon after sundown. We do nothing of the sort, so has the body clock reset itself?

We spend a large part of our waking hours in artificial light. Day invades night insidiously, and when work is done, relaxation involves a like set of amusements at home—TV or computer screen—and outdoors, bright lights keep the city swinging till dawn. Our shopping malls are crowded well past midnight.

Sleep deprivation, night shifts, and jet lag have been investigated repeatedly and the findings suggest a definite change in the circadian rhythm of appetite and satiation, with predictable metabolic consequences. These are special situations.

What about changes we now embrace as routine?

'Night hunger', the craving for food in the hours around bedtime is quite common. If we don't reach for that tantalizing snack, it leads to our lying sleepless till we raid the fridge. This has been related to high levels of ghrelin, but it is also a pattern that soon establishes itself as obesity. Similarly, 'sleep apnoea' is very common in obesity. There are the usual obvious physical reasons for this, the pressure of abdominal contents compressing the lungs and therefore reduced ventilation is the commonest. The converse has also been noticed equally. Sleep apnoea can lead to obesity, when sleep deprivation causes metabolic derangement.

It isn't the total hours of sleep that matter as much as the sleeping time being 'out of phase'.

Laboratory studies on normal subjects made to sleep twelve hours out of phase with their usual rhythm, showed low leptin levels, high blood sugar, and high levels of insulin. They also had 'diabetic' sugar values after a meal.

Recently, the secretion of melatonin, the hormone that regulates circadian rhythms, has been shown to be disrupted in diabetes. That is one more feature to suggest Metabolic Syndrome involves a gear shift in our circadian rhythms.

Charlie Chaplin made *Modern Times* in 1936. Eighty years later, the factory sequences in the movie seem to describe Digital India. If the struggle to survive wears a different face today, it is a struggle nonetheless.

Like the factory worker of the American Depression, middle-class Indians face the same helpless pressure exerted by the system. A 9-to-5 job means a fourteen-hour day, for the travails of getting to work can only be matched by the exhaustion of getting home. Unless we have the grand advantage of living close to our workplace, we commute. The exigencies of domesticity that precede the commute are just as tiring and the commute is always taxing. Noise, near suffocation in crowded buses and trains, interminable queues, and through all this the anxiety of being late.

Stress is so much a part of daily routine that it is a wonder we still continue to feel its oppression. At the same time, we accept it as a destined part of existence and do nothing to combat it *while it is happening*.

Yes, de-stressors are aplenty, beginning with that magical cup of green tea in office, to yogasana wherever you can manage mat space.

I find all this very unintelligent.

Why not refuse stress?

Oh yes, it can be done—environmental stress can be

refused by an active curiosity about our surroundings. We Indians are past masters in the art of conquering misery. We see it being done every day with humour, kindness and beauty in the most squalid and harsh surroundings.

Refusing emotional stress is much more difficult, and all of us bear this burden in today's India, with interpersonal communication largely reduced to emoticons.

Could stress contribute to our national obesity?

Take a look at what happens when I'm caught in a traffic jam, late for work. The noise is unbelievable. Everybody is honking, phones ring madly, quarrels heat up—my head's about to explode.

At this point, my hypothalamus unleashes two hormones. One whizzes to the adrenals and steps up production of adrenaline. The other raises blood pressure. Together, they activate the delicate Hypothalamus-Pituitary-Adrenal (H-P-A) axis which operates on negative feedback to release the stress hormone adrenaline to prepare the body for battle.

But it is only a traffic jam!

I don't need this biochemical response that stress has primed my body for. By now I'm awash with adrenaline. That raises my blood sugar. It elbows out insulin, even though I need it right now to utilize my breakfast smartly. My blood pressure is going through the roof. By the time I get to my appointment, I'm cramped from being behind the wheel for two hours. I'm exhausted—and it isn't yet 9.30 a.m.

I call for tea, and slump into my chair.

My tea arrives hot and syrupy, and with it, a packet of biscuits. Gosh, that was good!

Was it?

It wasn't hunger that called for that snack, it was stress.

Adrenaline's call for instant energy was translated into an urgent need for tea and biscuits. Not only is adrenaline orexogenic, it orders a specific menu—high fats and high sugar.

If the H-P-A axis operates entirely on negative feedback, then it should put its feet up after my snack.

But it also works via the reward system.

So, my as-yet-undigested breakfast received a top-up with tea and chocolate biscuits.

Wait—did I say *chocolate* biscuits?

Naturally, I skip lunch. A couple of chais, a hot samosa at four o'clock and I've powered through the evening. It's dark when I leave office. I grab a packet of biscuits against the long drive ahead.

A heavy dinner gets me dyspeptic, but I like something sweet after my Spartan fare—

Two hours later, battling heartburn, I ponder all the wrong decisions that led up to this moment. And to think it all started with that traffic jam!

Part 2

MATÉRIEL & METHODOLOGIES

Breakfast on the Street

The chaiwallah at the gate is taking a breather. He drops a fragrant handful of pounded ginger and cardamom into the boiling vat of tea. It has been cooking since dawn. Every hour or so he throttles a milk carton in a wristy grip. Customers look on approvingly as a white jet punctures the roiling tide of tea, knowing they will get their money's worth. His chai is nothing if not kadak. Each serving (Rs 10) is a little more than an ounce, a milky syrup astringent with tannins.

I recall a conversation I had three days ago with a loyal customer. It was 5.30 a.m., and he was getting his petrol, as he put it, before starting his autorickshaw for the day.

'This sits in the stomach like a stone,' he confided as he slurped an appreciative mouthful. 'And where else do you get chai as kadak, along with a paan on the ready, at this hour?'

A1 Paan, across the street, had been doing brisk business for the past half half-an-hour.

My friend admitted he didn't go in for A1's Specials at this hour.

'*Bas, normal paan hi theek hai*,' he said.

His next meal would be around 11 a.m.—if he was lucky. Otherwise, chai and paan held the day together till his 2 p.m. lunch break. He belched richly as he told me this, a ripe rumble that certified the chai as *ek number cheez*. The worst of rickshaw driving, he said, was magaj-maari, stress. It got his digestion all upset, so he was never without his tablets.

'Prescribed by your doctor?' I ventured

He spat derisively. 'Who's got time for doctors? Rascals! They charge fees, don't they? Whatever for? We still have to buy the medicines, don't we? The chemist tells all, sells all. *Paisa vasool.*'

His pocket pharmacy was predictable: two sorts of antacid, H_2 inhibitors, proton-pump inhibitors (PPIs), eight kinds of tablets in all—the wishful pharmacopoeia of acid-dyspeptic disease.

'Do you eat all this every day?' I asked.

'Most days, just the pink ones. Some days are so bad, I just swallow the whole handful.'

'What's it like today?'

He grimaced. 'Normal.'

That's a delicately nuanced word. Synonymous with *usual*, it defines unusual as *ab*normal. But it also reflects acceptance and resignation to suffering beyond relief, and often enough, beyond belief. Snafu.

He picked out three pink tablets and munched on them with distaste.

'Keeps me going,' he shrugged.

That's another phrase I'm getting used to. On the street you've got to keep going.

What keeps us going?

Breakfast, to begin with.

8.20 a.m. on a Thursday morning. I am out to discover what my street eats for breakfast. Surely breakfast is the last meal that springs to mind when you think of street food? One more instance of how a preconceived notion can blinker observation. Most early workers, if they breakfast at all, grab a bite off the street

Eight is late. Early breakfasters, long replete, are halfway through a busy morning.

Across the road, a fruit vendor is setting out his counter with an air of hopelessness.

Next to him, there is more action.

A four-burner stove makes a merry blaze beneath a venerable kadhai. Its puddle of oil is even more ancient, turbid and viscous with age. An early harvest is already sweating: a clutch of onion pakodas, a few amorphous bondas, three dented samosas. Perhaps they are leftovers awaiting resurrection when the oil begins to smoke—but I don't get to see that.

Something more compelling grabs my attention.

Kids!

Suddenly there are children everywhere, erupting on pavements, oozing out of dark crevices between shopfronts, pouring down the road from the tenements uphill. The oldest about eleven, the youngest six or seven. Upper Primary, Class 1 to 7. Despite their noisy cheer, they look wan and unbreakfasted.

I am surprised to see them rush to the general store. It isn't ready for business yet. The owner, fresh from his bath, wet towel plastered to his chest, waves an arati through the dim interior, tinkling a bell to inaugurate the day before switching on the lights.

I line up to buy a cake of soap I don't need, and investigate the buzz.

Each knot of kids has an older boy as spokesman. There are very few girls around, unless you count trusting little sisters. Older girls swing past nonchalant. They are just as wan and unbreakfasted, but clearly, store invasion isn't their thing.

I am reminded of a long-ago morning when I walked my six-year-old daughter home from school. She skipped ahead uncaring as someone called out her name with increasing desperation. When I protested, her reaction was a jaw-dropper: 'It's just a *boy*, Daddy. Ignore him!'

These boys at the store cannot be ignored.

Each spokesman, empowered to spend five bucks, is watched lynx-eyed by his gang.

Biscuits? Cream or sada? Chocolate? Toffee?

'Get on with it!' The shopkeeper, shivering in his damp clothes, is testy.

Biscuits win hands down: a five-buck pack gets you one each. The kids scamper off, rejoicing.

That's it?

One biscuit to jumpstart the day?

Rubbish, I scold myself. Surely their mothers made certain their stomachs weren't empty when they left home. Or did they?

I trail two boys and a girl. They are dragging their feet. Their legs are practically Euclidean lines—length without breadth, their backs bowed under heavy bags. Just past the bus stop, the girl drops her bag and settles down in a doorway to stretch her legs. The boys hesitate, then join her silently. Their misery is a visible fug around them. They are wrapped in an intimacy of exhaustion and woe, it is their language of being.

What grief or loss has robbed their faces of day? My helplessness kills me.

A cumulus of egrets settles on the dying rain-tree across the road.

The girl breaks the trance. 'White birds!' Her sweet voice is wistful, almost Dickensian.

The moment is Dickensian too. The three small faces morph from sadness into wonder as the birds take off. Laughter rings out brave and carefree. The older brother picks up the girl's bag and walks ahead. They trot behind, holding hands.

The fancier eateries are still shut. Amritsari Kulcha Junction (its signboard a burning promise of chillies red and green), Chilly & Onion (Chinese & More: A Family Dining Experience) and the new swank ice-cream store which flaunts the hottest selling line this festive week—Ganesha's

Favourite Flavour—Boondi and Modak Ice-cream. These won't swing into action till lunch time,

The King of Deep Fry is open for business even though its gargantuan kadhai, surgically scrubbed to a dazzle, is still upended on a cold stove.

Hot Chips is a chain, and the name explains itself. An added warning announces: All Snacks South Indian Taste. This kiosk has been around for the last fifteen years and I have often watched chips being fried by the ton, impressed by two observations. The oil is never allowed to smoke or thicken. The chips are never 'oily'—they leave no more than the veriest trace of grease—on the fingertip, on tissue paper, and most importantly for me, on the tongue.

The two boys at the counter look as if they've just tumbled out of bed, eyes still gummy with sleep. The only customer, a middle-aged woman demanding potato chips, clucks impatiently, 'Get some tea, maybe your brains will start working then.' They smile good-humouredly and serve her. They shake out a sample of tapioca chips for me to taste.

Each woody frill is delicate as a pencil shaving, crisp and nutty, just faintly salted. There are more aggressive editions, rouged with chilli powder, or curled beneath a lethal impasto of green chillies and herbs.

The shop opens at 8 a.m. and closes at 11 p.m., with no break for lunch or tea. Frying begins at 10 a.m., and they are generally done by late afternoon.

The shelves gleam with light, a study of the spectrum between 570 and 590 nm. The entire gamut of yellow, stretched between green and orange. To my right, the faint lime green of chilli- and coriander-stained crisps. To my left, the belligerent tincture of red chilli. And everything between has the warm glow of carotenoids. Turmeric, yes, but also the gold of besan, the apricot blush of jackfruit and banana.

What about tartrazine? Sunset yellow?

The boys don't know the chemical handles, but are alert

to food colouring. It is a question they get asked often these days. Their answer is pat: 'Only natural. Turmeric, red and green chillies, coriander.'

The far wall is crammed with packaged snacks. The dichotomy is obvious. Traditional murukku in subdued yellows, and cornflour fritters in lurid yellow, orange and green. No hotshot machines here, the perfect circles of murukku and chakri simply show off expertise in an ancient Indian food tech: extrusion. The boys need their breakfast, so I'm not going to ask them to show me their moulds and pressers. Perhaps another time.

Ganesh and Nagappa are from Salem, where most kids sign up with food chains like this one. They learn on the job. It takes less than a week to perfect their skills.

Really?

'It took me ten days,' Ganesh confesses.

'One week, me.' Nagappa grins.

'We keep at it till we get it right,' Ganesh adds.

No mean skill, as any home cook will certify.

They use up 14–15 litres of refined oil a day, and ten to fifteen sacks of potatoes, for potato chips remain their hottest item. How much of that do they sell? About 10–15 kg a day.

How does that compare with other stores?

Not too well, Ganesh admits. 'But with an upgrade—'

His gesture of helplessness is much more eloquent. There's a flash of something deeper than pain in his eyes. He is looking at an endless procession of tomorrows balancing 10 kg of fried goods against 14 litres of oil—where's the escape?

What about the other snacks?

Chivda here goes by the name of Mixture, but Ganesh assures me they make every sort. Garlic & Chilli moves the fastest.

Nagappa scoops up a generous sample for me, but I pass.

The potato chip customer who has stayed on to breakfast commandeers it eagerly.

'Get your breakfast now,' she urges Nagappa who is stifling a yawn.

'Not yet, maybe in an hour,' he responds.

And what will he have for breakfast? Chips? Chivda? Murukku?

'Tea and a banana.'

The women salvaging plastic from the dump are from Ganesh's neck of the woods. I know most of them by name. Already deep in the rhythm of work, they are not to be disturbed now. They start at 6 and break for tea at eleven. Just tea. What about breakfast? They've eaten at home at five-thirty. Hot idlis or pazhedu, fermented rice, a village staple. Samosa and vada? The suggestion earns a scornful look. Just– fluff!

Up the road, the only eatery of significance is Kabab Korner, and that's strictly evening trade.

On to the main road then.

Already there's an arterial throb of buses and trucks. Drivers grit their molars against the steady infusion of pedestrians, and the madcap spatter of children late for school. Kids scamper off to safety. Drivers rev up for heart attacks and strokes.

The hospital is the main road's only punctuation. Here the rhythm alters, and not, as one might expect, into urgency. Quite the contrary. It becomes leisured and ruminant.

I notice people on the street who don't seem to be going anywhere. Their sole intent seems simply to be here. They are not loitering; they are very focussed in their intent to linger on the street.

Who are they?

A familiar lot to hospital staff, they are the weary,

cramped, irritated, anxious, and well nigh broke but healthy population of the hospital. The friends and relations who sustain the sick. Their incessant buzz of cheer, gossip and reproach is the quickest aid to recovery. The sick get well from sheer desperation after a day or two of enduring them.

Conviviality around the sick bed has an etiquette all its own. It combines all the familiarities of a family reunion with the scandalous thrills of a masquerade. The patient is just the catalyst, and once the action has taken off, can be safely ignored. The talk is all about *finding out*, with a generous pinch of telling-all in the most circuitous way possible.

An incredible charge of curiosity enlivens the smallest detail. Epics can be spun out of IV drips. Ancestors resurrected with physical horrors intact. Pregnancies back-tracked to their dubious origins (dates are matched). Diarrhoeas are enumerated, darkly predictive of the child's dismal future. A rich vein of humour glistens through every tragedy, blackly subversive, drawing an unwilling smile from the fierce Ward Sister herself.

It takes tremendous energy to keep this mill churning, and friends and relations require hourly infusions. There is only so much one can pack in a standard tiffin-carrier, and, let's face it, where's the thrill in eating 'home food' in hospital?

The patient's own meal tray is quickly sampled and rejected. The canteen's repertoire is just as quickly exhausted (same cook)—besides it's shameful how they expect you to pay for snacks even though you're meeting a big fat bill—

And this 8 a.m. jaunt—the first foray after a cramped night on a corridor bench, bitten raw by mosquitoes, jolted awake by someone else's dying relative *twice*, staring at the dark for hours after the body's trundled past—this is serious stuff.

Mere breakfast cannot suffice. This calls for triage. And where else do you turn, but to the street?

The hub is easily spotted. A food cart, invisible behind a wall of impatient customers. With some dedicated manoeuvring, I find a station at the chef's elbow. A strapping young man in a green t-shirt, he's at this moment raising a dripping mound of bhajiyas out of a smoking kadhai. To my left, the sous is hard at work chopping an onion.

I'm impressed by the economy: of space, of utensils, of implements, of movement. Of speech.

The cart is as intelligently assembled as a surgical trolley. Everything has its appointed place, carefully restored after each use with near-ritualistic precision.

All this minimalism works because of sheer expertise. The leisurely pace is deceptive. It hides a ruthless efficiency. When the sous cuts his finger, he continues chopping till that onion is done.

The chopping board is a miracle in itself, an oblong strip just an inch wide, a one-onion affair. The diced onion is off the board and the next under the knife in a twinkling.

The counter's tin top is swabbed of crumbs, a sheet of newspaper tucked beneath the chopping board for the next batch of onions.

Pankaj, the sous chef, isn't too particular about his knife work; a coarse chop suffices.

Sunil, the chef, is now readying the next offering for the demonic kadhai.

Smoke billows, blue, acrid, quickly staunched as batter hits the oil.

This is the most popular item on the menu.

Sunil calls it a cutlet.

Thirty years ago, my college canteen gave it a different name—Bread Bhajiya. Two slices of bread slammed against last night's leftovers, dipped in besan and fried entire. You could eat it crisped by a second frying twelve hours later as well. At teatime it sold even better as Sandwich Fry.

Sunil's opus is the very same dish, but the stuffing is fresh and very aromatic. A spicy meld of potato, Pankaj's onions, and a shovel of green stuff guaranteed to sting.

The sandwiches are gargantuan triangles. The boys use large loaves of sliced bread, two slices to the plate. This is a breakfast item, Sunil explains. They go through seventeen large loaves every morning. That's about 170 plates.

The cutlets come up now, crisp and golden. A quick shake to rid them of oil and they are sent out to waiting customers. Served on clean steel trays with neat puddles of sambar, sauce, and a choice of chutneys, you can't do better at twenty bucks, can you?

Oh yes you can, I decide, as Sunil hauls a 10-kg steel dabba on to the counter. A cloud of urad wells out. Batter for medu vadai, ready spiked with jeera and garlic. He drops in fistfuls of chopped ginger, coriander, green chillies, curry leaves. It is a treat to watch Sunil shape the vadais, each one a perfect dimpled cushion. Twelve of them slide off his slat-like palm for the first batch.

'Eight kilos of urad a day, one-and-a-half tins of oil.'

A tin of oil is 15 litres, do the math.

He is a skilled cook, but old habits die hard. The oil, fast thickening to a sludge, is simply topped up. It is a 2-litre kadhai. Modest, no more than a dozen medu vadais per batch. The vadais have puffed up beautifully now, and Sunil turns them over to crisp.

The boys are from Kanpur—though, admittedly, this is Bombay cuisine; the same stuff sells well in Kanpur too.

Daal vada, the next on the menu, comes ready ground in another giant dabba. Sunil does a quick dice of palak, sweeps in Pankaj's onions, and a medley of green stuff, then gives it all a good stir.

This is second-most popular item, he tells me.

The other frivolities—vada pao, onion pakodas—imprisoned in a glass case, are evidently just display.

'Evening snacks,' Pankaj explains loftily. 'That stuff's okay for evening, but for breakfast, it must be cutlet and vada.'

'What about idli?'

'Sometimes, not every day.'

Sunil packs two plump and crisp vadai for me. Plastic packets of sambar and chutney neatly knotted, and a warm invitation to come again completes the transaction.

Sunil has the expansive gravitas of a true plutocrat—which he is. The boys also own all the ancillary businesses that power this breakfasts. From the dry provisions, the potatoes and vegetables, to the mill that grinds 10 kg of each kind of batter every day, it is all in the family.

'I just want people to be happy, fill their stomachs with good food on a twenty buck note,' Sunil says.

Judging from the aroma of the vadai crackling in my package, he seems to have succeeded brilliantly.

The brain maybe mostly fat, but it doesn't like discussions about this. Reading about fat leaves my brain benumbed, and not a little resentful. After the last few pages, I guess yours must be too.

We've squelched through the plethora of information about dietary fat. How do we choose in the kitchen?

Fat multi-tasks to serve up a delicious meal.

It *cooks* food in many different ways: deep fry, sauté, bake, broil.

It *flavours* food as tempering in a tadka, or garnish in a dressing.

It *textures* food to increase its sensuous appeal by smoothing emulsions, as in ice-cream or gravy.

We slather it mindlessly on every food in the simple faith that it *improves taste*.

And we have such a wide array of fats—how do we pick the right one for the job?

To deep fry, we usually pick oil.

Few homes today use traditional oils—mustard, coconut, sesame—for deep frying.

Most of us rely on 'refined oils'.

Actually, we overlook the oil—we just don't want it around in the finished product.

We need something that will leave a chip or a chakli crisp and non-greasy. The food has its own flavour—we don't want the oil for that.

Generally, our oil of choice has a high Omega-6 content.

Often, a vanaspati* is used instead of oil. This means more trans fats. It also means a crisper, lighter product on your plate.

Most homes now don't use vanaspati. Also, most people tell me they *never deep fry.*

What they *don't* tell me, unless I ask, is how much of deep-fried foods they eat. True, they don't cook them at home. Why should they, when the market is bursting with crisp, flaky delicacies so hygienically packed?

Just one hint: most commercial crisps are deep fried in vanaspati, and are therefore, very high in trans fats.

Sauté is the elegant term for frying anything very quickly in very little, very hot fat. Flavour is important here for two reasons.

---

*From the Sanskrit, *vanaspati* literally means 'Lord of the Forest' and refers to the plant kingdom. *Vanaspati* is also the Indian slang for vanaspati ghee or margarine, hydrogenated vegetable cooking oil, used as the cheaper substitute for ghee and butter. In India, vanaspati ghee is usually made from palm oil.

First, and most importantly, fat dissolves the volatile oils in spices to offer the accord which accounts for the 'masala taste'. This allows flavour to infuse through the food being cooked.

The second reason is that the flavour of the oil itself is integral to the dish.

This is usually where the maximum amount of fat is used in cooking the meal.

It could be oil or ghee or a mixture of both.

Traditional oils are in play here, for that authentic flavour.

While the finished dish may have a succulent gravy, sautéing is usually the first step towards achieving this.

Tawa roasting of spices is the alternative method for this step. This takes about 25 per cent or less fat than is needed to sauté.

Baking incorporates fat into the raw ingredients. The food is cooked in fat as it heats up slowly and the fat is completely absorbed. A successfully baked product should not be greasy to the touch.

Traditionally, baking employs animal fats: butter, cream, milk, curds, cheese, eggs, lard. These are all saturated fats.

After 1911, when hydrogenated oils entered the market, cooks discovered that they baked even better. Hydrogenated oil, margarine or vanaspati, was the fat of choice for commercial baking till we discovered the dangers of trans fats. Since then, oils and zero-trans margarines have ruled. The home baker follows this lead.

Baked foods (except bread) contain more fat than foods cooked any other way. A fluffy balushahi that melts on the tongue has only half the fat contained in a modest slice of plain, depressingly heavy cake.

A good rule of thumb: the 'lighter' a baked product feels, the more fat it contains.

All Indian cuisine relies on tempering, tadka, for that final burst of flavour to complete the dish. This garnish usually consists of aromatics: oil seeds, spices, daals, herbs. The technique releases the volatiles at a high temperature, and the hot fat dissolves them rapidly as it is slid onto the cooked dish. Very little fat is needed to accomplish this—but who ever notices that?

Dressing a cooked dish with cold oil is used in some traditional Indian dishes, yes, but this is a byword in Western cuisine where the sparkle of the fresh, the crisp, the raw, is usually tutored into sullen conformity with olive oil.

Texturing food with fat renders it creamy.

In Indian cuisine, dairy in the form of beaten curds or cream is the usual additive. In Western cuisine, it is usually butter, cream or egg yolks. The mouthfeel of creaminess is irresistible to the Western palate. We Indians are a tad hesitant over most emulsions, except ice-cream!

Oil can be used to achieve emulsions too.

So, if you tot up these different techniques of using fat in your own kitchen, you'll have a fair idea of the fats you use in *cooking*.

There are also many uncooked fats we consume at home: all dairy products, nuts and seeds.

Those apart, you can take it for granted that all pickles, sauces and dips are full of fat.

A day later, at the same hour, I'm on the terrace, transcribing my impressions of breakfast on the street.

Dazzling sun, welcome after a week of lowering skies, and the air lilts with birdsong. Butterflies and dragonflies dip and zoom to trap the sun in their wings. Treetops reveal parrots still in déshabille. I watch them preen and elegantly dress for the day. Kites circle low enough for me to see their bastard wings. Fat doves flutter and strut on the parapet, dazzling rhinestone collars around their necks.

The street seems very far away.

Cooking smells float up to my balcony from the other flats in my building and I recognize my neighbours by the accord.

Hot oil, pappadam.

Hot oil, garlic.

Hot oil, jeera and mustard.

Hot ghee, curry leaves, jeera, asafoetida.

A sudden waft of paratha followed by a slap of overheated oil.

That is a lot of oil heating up.

And it's just 'Home Food'—a garnish, a sauté, a mere dab of oil.

If you want to see oil in all its glory, 'Outside Food', already a-sizzle on the pavement at this early hour, makes a braver display.

Outside food trades on the miracles of fat.

Deep fry the day!

What does it mean exactly, to deep fry?

The technique is practically fool-proof: drop something squishy into hot oil and up it comes, crunchy and golden.

The conspirators in this coup, batter and filling, aren't very impressive by themselves.

For squish, there is potato. Elsewhere it maybe little more than a globus of starch, but it is India's uber tuber.

(What's that? Of course it is 100 per cent Indian! It is our national vegetable, isn't it? Peruvian—pah! Our Vedas were powered on aloo dum when South America was still a soggy strip of Gondwanaland. Gondwana? Google it, you'll find it is somewhere in Madhya Pradesh, or maybe Odisha. Oh yes, Peru itself was once Indian, most definitely, not just the potato.)

Survival food?

Sure.

With us, survival is an art form, and nothing lends itself to self-expression quite as willingly as the potato, so lavish in plenitude and practically impossible to insult. Good-humoured to the point of imbecility, its blandness is 'adjustment' incarnate. It can mother, with equal fortitude, brain-dead rozi roti or extreme cuisine.

So here's our old reliable, steamed to perfection, raising a friendly bleb of enquiry on its khaki jacket: *what shall we do today?*

Let us turn the potato into a demagogue, a rabble-rouser, a polyglot that gets its point across no matter where.

Look what happens when you turn a potato into a vada.

Call it what you will, vada, bonda, or even bombé, its appeal is equally irrational and irresistible. It is an unreasonable expectation.

How can a wodge of stodge in a splatter of batter ever find its way to fame?

Ah, but when it struts onto your plate, the vada is a very different animal. Breaking past its polite dermis, it erupts as a volcanic surge of eloquence—texture, aroma, flavour, taste—to completely disavow its forlorn beginnings.

This transformation is brought about by the quickest, laziest, most ubiquitous cooking method—deep frying.

Ball it, batter it, drop it.

Wait till it stops sizzling.

Retrieve, drain.

Slap on a dollop of chutney—voila!

A no-brainer, right?

Something any cook at the end of her tether might invent.

And how intelligent the transformation!

So where is the genius in it?

First, the potato is steamed. That educates it a tad: the starch turns faintly glassy—it has begun to 'gelatinize'. Water has entered the starch molecules, allowing them to swell up. The cell walls have not ruptured; they've just been forced apart. The cellulose has become more digestible. The protein has coagulated.

This is a potato so ready to be eaten, it seems a pity to maul it. But it is mashed thoughtlessly. It subsides into a mealy cumulus, silky to the fingertip and faintly sweet. In the racy company of onions, ginger, herbs and spices, over the next few minutes it acquires some piquancy, but that's just a surface skill. Its innocent heart is still bland starch.

Pop it into hot oil and you know what you'll get: a greasy blob of dejected glue.

So it teams up with batter.

The batter forms a protective shell that keeps the potato from getting gluey as it goes back into the oil. Although it's been engaged only as a lowly buffer, the batter's chemical smarts earn it star status.

The standard batter is besan (chickpea flour to you), with the occasional dash of rice flour. Season it, spice it, whisk it with cold water.

The perfect batter is what a cook recognizes as 'dropping consistency'.

Non-cooks can test it on a flat surface.

It falls as a blob, not a splatter.

Tip the plate and it takes off at an amble, looking over its shoulder as it spreads.

It smears rather than streaks.

Any thicker, and your vada will be a pachyderm.

Any thinner will get you a vada in greasy off-shoulder déshabille.

The oil in the kadhai for deep frying should be at 160 to 180°C. Lower temperatures will yield a soggy and greasy product. Higher temperatures will char the food.

As the vada hits hot oil, heat is transferred into it. Water in the batter heats up, boils and evaporates with an audible sizzle. Oil enters the pores left by water vapour.

This transfers more heat to the centre and the starch of the potato begins to gelatinize, and changes the lumpy filling into a silky lava.

Meanwhile, the batter is changing rapidly too as it loses water. It hardens and crisps up.

At this point, the kadhai sends out signals.

The first signal is auditory. The sizzle.

The second signal is olfactory.

A lungful of roasty toasty aromas waft right across the road. It doesn't matter what's frying, the aroma promises endless delight.

The third signal is visual. Bobbing in the oil are gold hemispheres. The sight taps into a basic human lust, call it beauty, call it greed, but we ache to hold it.

The fourth signal—and it takes some self-control NOT to react immediately to it—is tactile. The texture—crisp, fragile, flaky, tender. (How come oily is overlooked?)

The fingertips delighted, the mouth awaits its turn, sluiced with anticipatory juices, impatient for a bite.

I said it before and I'll say it again—no matter what's being fried, the signals are all the same. It is all in the batter.

Needless to say, frying at a lower temperature won't broadcast any of these interesting signals, so the hot oil has something to do with it too.

The high temperature frees sugars and amino acids in the batter to begin one of the most important biochemical changes in cooking.

The reaction between amino acids and sugars produces both colour and aroma. A hundred years ago, this reaction excited Louis-Camille Maillard, a medical student in France. He published a paper—'Action Des Acides Aminés Sur Les Sucres; Formation Des Mélanoïdines Par Voie Méthodique.'*

*L.C. Maillard, 'Action des acides aminé's sur les sucres: Formation des mélanoidines par voie méthodique,' Compte-rendu de l'Académie des sciences, 1912, pp. 66–68.

This was the first of many in which Maillard referred to the change as 'my reaction'. He published more papers that referred to this change. Not surprisingly, it became known, quite early in his career, as the Maillard Reaction.

Every foodie knows this fancy name for the change that turns food red, brown, crisp, and liberates all those toasty aromas.

The chemical steps of a Maillard Reaction have been unremittingly studied over the century since it was first described, and surprises are still rife.

At first the research was prompted by curiosity in the transformation itself—why does high temperature turn soggy food into a crisp, flavourful and aromatic delight?

Once the basic chemistry was explained, interest grew in the resulting compounds that do so much to improve food quality, and it became all about enhancing these attributes.

Yes, food looks, smells and tastes more exciting because the Maillard Reaction releases dozens of interesting new molecules. But what happens to the food itself?

Sugars which are oligosaccharides (like raffinose, sucrose and stachynose) undergo hydrolysis and are converted into glucose, fructose and galactose, to make the food taste sweeter.

At high temperatures, amino acids like lysine, histidine and arginine are destroyed, and this makes the food less nutritious.

It is not all bad news.

Chemicals released by the reaction, Maillard Reaction Products (MRPs) are anti-oxidants.

Anybody who reads food labels in supermarkets knows all about this magic word.

Anti-oxidants promise true believers immortality at a not very distant date. Skeptics, please keep reading this book!

The actual value of the anti-oxidants in MRPs is, naturally, being fiercely debated, as anything that might threaten the food industry will certainly be.

Think of it, how can something so delectably crisp be bad for you?

Some MRPs make up a group called Advanced Glycation End-Products. With an apt acronym—AGE, these chemicals are being held responsible for cardiovascular illnesses, and less catastrophically, for ageing.

Without the Maillard Reaction, vadas will be soft and greasy. And more to the point for the vendor of these delights—unsold.

Out on the street, the kadhai goes into overdrive at peak hour.

Now something new happens.

Successive batches of cutlets, vadas and bhajiyas have sweated out enough water from the batter for the oil to undergo a change called hydrolysis. This lowers the smoking point of the oil and also makes it thicker.

As frying continues, as the temperature climbs and the oil thickens, the Maillard Reaction intensifies, and gives rise to a compound called *acrylamide*.

This sounds more like a plastic than anything edible, and, it should come as no shock to discover that late-morning vadas carry a hefty shot of acrylamide.

And acrylamide is toxic to brain cells.

It is, also, a credible carcinogen.

The sad truth is that acrylamide is quite easy to produce in the kitchen of the very careful and informed cook—all it takes is deep frying in very hot oil for very long.

Deep frying what?

Er...batter.

Any kind of flour will shake out the requisite free sugars and amino acids, some more than others. Besan, chick-pea flour, has a very high content of asparagine, a starter molecule for acrylamide.

Our late morning vada has also absorbed a lot of this gunky oil. It is now rich in toxic aldehydes and alkyl benzenes.

So it does begin to look as if every vat of boiling oil on the street is a conspiracy against its devoted customers.

Or, is this needless panic?

Haven't we been gorging on deep-fried delights for millennia?

What has changed, so suddenly, now?

Have we changed?

Did we gorge on deep-fried delights first thing in the morning even ten years ago, leave alone a millennium ago?

Haven't we changed?

That's what happens to the vada—but what happens to you and me when faced with these Golden Globe exquisites?

In one word they look—appetizing.

What exactly does 'appetizing' mean?

It is 8 a.m. and eighteen-year-old Shalini alights from a bus.

She left home at 6 after a hasty cup of tea. A mad sprint for the bus, a scramble for the fast train, and now, after a long wait in the queue, another bus ride. She still has a ten-minute walk ahead to her college gates, if she's to make the first lecture on time.

Breakfast?

You're kidding, right?

Across the road, a food stall is frying the first batch of batata vadas. The kadhai wafts a powerful lot of aromatics.

Shalini turns, quite without volition.

It is a moment worthy of Kalidasa.

She hurries forward determinedly, but the thorn is just as persistent. She stops for one more glance over her shoulder, catches a glimpse of the vadas as they emerge from the oil in all their golden allure, and simply cannot look away. If only the vendor wouldn't persist in shaking those vadas in the air for quite so long—

But he does, and the seduction is complete.

Trapped in a chemical rush, Shalini's brain forswears that geology lecture.

One desperate glance at her watch, a quick check in her purse for cash, and Shalini dashes across the road.

Ten minutes later, Shalini gobbles the last morsel of vada, totally unconscious of certain marvellous changes that have occurred within her. She doesn't know, for instance, that the moment she took her first bite—before she registered the hit of chilli and garlic, even before she had actually tasted the mouthful—her intestines were already hard at work, pushing out the right set of chemicals to digest the vada.

Already?

Before she had swallowed the first morsel?

Shalini's intestines knew what the vada would contain, knew its chemical composition down to the final molecule. Okay, maybe not down to the ultimate nuance of spice, but the basic building blocks seem an open secret.

How could her intestines, those coils happily concealed in her hot-pink kurti, possibly know? Even food chemists, who spend all day squinting at molecules, do not.

The answer is in that first delicious mouthful that is so tasty.

Shalini's taste receptors are more than pleasure sensors. They are dazzlingly sentient, they locate each note in every pleasant tune.

So, while Shalini's mouth hums with the familiar pentatonic scale of salt, sweet, tart, bitter, umami, there are grace notes science is just beginning to discover.

The brain receives exceptional biochemical information encoded in these gustatory gamaka. It learns the exact state of the oil smoking in the kadhai. It learns about the proteins in the crust, the sugars in the melting potato, the fatty acids jostling their way into the vada. Naturally, it lets the stomach know.

Geographically, the gastrointestinal (GI) tract is miles away from the 'tasting area' of the brain—and the GI tract is pretty long in itself—25 feet even in our petite Shalini.

Conversations, therefore, need very quick messaging.

You could dismiss that as 'involuntary', as we've done for a century or more. Or, you could wake up to a newer intelligence.

This intelligence announces itself as Shalini is halfway through her snack.

Things begin to get complicated at this point.

As the first morsel of vada sloshes around in the stomach, tiny particles are sent on ahead into the small intestine.

As the amuse bouche arrives in the upper ileum, something rather shocking happens. The cells in the intestinal lining taste the vada.

Yes, you read that right.

Imagine having tastebuds studding twenty feet of slither.

The Tamil idiom for a persnickety diner is naaku neellam, having a very long tongue.

Even if that didn't extend to twenty feet, it yet carries a grain of very literal truth.

The tastebuds of the small intestine are vociferous critics.

A terse review of that first morsel might read: nice, but nasty.

And unlike those long-tongued critics who merely disparage the food of others, intestinal taste receptors act on their convictions. They send back a health warning: *Watch out, fat overload!*

Shalini, who has now also ordered a plate of cutlets, does not hear this.

Or perhaps she does, but can't interpret it.

That warning didn't sound in her brain as a consciously

worded thought, but she should have received it just the same.

The warning was sent around in so many ways to so many places—by nerve impulses to the stomach and intestine, by chemical messengers in the bloodstream to just about everywhere, and particularly to the brain.

The stomach and intestine read the message at once in all its simplicity because it translated into a shout: ENOUGH!

The intestinal lining oozed out chemicals that ordered the brain to 'feel full', the stomach to stop churning, and look for its HOUSE FULL signboard.

Meanwhile, the morsel has reached the lower intestine, and the food critics here are as mean as Gordon Ramsay force-fed vegan for a week. The chemicals they produce don't stop at a gentle suggestion to slow down. They simply slam on the brakes.

The 'ileal brake' is the body's hard-wired defence against greed—perhaps even against obesity. Once it is activated, you feel stuffed.

Before she starts on her first crisp triangle of cutlet, Shalini is already feeling full, but somewhere in her brain is this picture of the stomach as a howling abyss. Those two small vadas have disappeared into its vacuum without a trace. They were vanquished in a couple of bites each. In terms of volume how can they possibly have filled her stomach?

So Shalini's jaw ignores her tightening midriff and powers on.

An hour later, Shalini finds herself nodding through the lecture.

Coffee?

Great idea.

Was it?

Shalini skips lunch. She's feeling listless and tired by afternoon.

A hit of kadak chai before the long haul home.

She's ravenous when she gets home. Biscuits, chips, multifarious farsan, tea, fruit juice. Nothing seems to quell the raging fire in her stomach.

She stares at her dinner in distaste, gets into a fight with her pesky brother, and leaves the room in tears.

'I just don't get it,' her mother worries. 'The poor child eats next to nothing and still puts on so much weight.'

'Don't fuss, she isn't fat, just healthy,' says her dad.

But Shalini, now sobbing in the dark, is just as puzzled as her mother.

She falls asleep worrying, and wakes up at midnight. The sleeping house feels peaceful, her bed is cozy, Shalini needs just a little something to ease herself back to sleep.

She reaches for the secret stash in her bag and finds a bar of chocolate. It is a big bar, sixteen squares. Shalini goes through eight of them before she falls asleep again.

You might dismiss Shalini as just another greedy person. That would not only be cruel, it would be scientifically wrong.

Like most overweight people, Shalini is resentful of well-meant and utterly pointless advice. She just knows nothing works.

You could console her with more meaningless stuff: genetic, familial, puppy fat.

Even chat her up on ghrelin and leptin.

Anything to assure her it's not her fault.

Everybody who loves her—and she's adorable, so the list is very long—rushes to reassure her how beautiful and glamourous she is.

And that just makes her gnash her teeth.

She knows she's beautiful and glamourous, dammit, which eighteen-year-old doesn't?

That's the last thing on her mind. She's worried about the way she's feeling.

Not exactly sick, no.

But low.

That about describes it.

She won't talk about it to her best friend. Every second person she knows is depressed.

First thing in the morning, Shalini decides on wellness big time. She surfs the net for a suitable gym. And while she's about that, finishes the rest of that bar of chocolate.

Shalini's street breakfast was 350 calories. With another 50 from a shot of syrupy kadak chai, that's a good whack of energy to start the day.

Or is it?

What does that term '400 calories' mean to your body?

What does it translate into, as your day progresses?

More than half of those calories came from oil.

People who aren't reading this book might protest. 'Oh, but that's not fat, is it? What's the difference between oil and fat?'

The most memorable answer comes from an eight-year-old who explained, 'Oil is what we eat, fat is what we are.'

Ouch.

Fat is what we are.

India, home of perpetual hunger, leads the world in obesity.

And, paradoxically, we have more hungry Indians than ever before.

Shalini was hungry the whole day after that 400-calorie breakfast. It did fill Shalini's stomach but she did not notice.

Why didn't she?

Why was she deaf to the body's signals?

This book is an attempt to understand that.

Before we listen to someone else, why not give one's own self a hearing?

What does the body feel about what we eat?

That is such a latitudinous question.

While genetic and environmental factors compel a highly individualistic response, our bodies still follow a species blueprint.

So how does the body respond to food?

This posits a separation between the physical body and the perceived self.

Does our body respond to food in a manner totally different from how we do?

Could this be true?

The Love Song of Lunch

Within half an hour of being chewed and swallowed, lunch is unrecognizable. It is a sour mush sloshing about in the stomach. Now and then, small doses trickle into the intestine, a tasting menu that charges twenty feet of digestive surface into readiness.

Digestion is a terrible gastronomic come down. Fine dining is reduced to primitive stuff, to biochemistry.

No matter how sophisticated its earlier guise, everything is now sorted into three groups: carbohydrate, protein, or fat.

Each group is commandeered by a set of chemicals. These enzymes will convert the large, unwieldy molecules into smaller travel-friendly forms.

Destination?

To any of the trillions of body cells—but we are tracking the food trail to the adipocyte. Surprisingly, it is not just fatty acids in that particular queue.

If the digestive tract were nothing more than a very long, very tedious, transit lounge, what a waste of space! A stomach like a tote bag and then miles of hose, all just to queue up a small meal?

Actually, the gut is more than a waiting area—it is an intelligence-processing unit as well. The gut lining contains an entire universe of microbes which not only interact with the waiting contents, but also tweet information through nerve endings and local chemicals to make up a complex intelligence network, the Gut-Brain-Axis.

But don't let that distract you, let's get back into queue.

The food has been organized into simple sugars (from carbohydrates), amino acids (from proteins), and fatty acids (from fats).

These simple-minded molecules are lined up against the intestinal wall, ready to board.

While we wait, check out their antecedents.

The sugars came from carbohydrates—rice, roti, daal, potato.

The amino acids from proteins in chicken, daal, and a smattering from rice and wheat.

This was a restaurant lunch. That guarantees a rush of fatty acids from the very large quantity of oil in the vegetables, chicken curry and, certainly, from the glistening biryani. The visible film of oil is merely a surface feature. Much more has been absorbed into the food itself. A very modest appraisal would be 2 tablespoons of oil.

The lunch deconstructed, reads:

70 gm carbohydrate

10 gm protein

30 gm fat

280 + 40 + 270 = 590 calories, a hefty whack of energy, with nearly 50 per cent sourced from fat.

Cooking oil is a triglyceride which needs to be broken down into free fatty acids and glycerol.

Within the body, fats and oils and their products of digestion are collectively called lipids.

While I was still chewing, fat digestion had already begun. The thousands of glands in my mouth sweated out minuscule droplets of the chemical that breaks down lipids. This enzyme is a lipase.

The gut has different editions of lipase, and that oral lipase is only the blurb.

The stomach has a better lipase, a paperback, good for a browse. It's also handy for making a quick resumé, and trickling that into the intestine as a flier. This happens very early, while the meal has just about begun, a tasting menu which gears up the gut for action.

The duodenum, sensing fat, releases a double-barreled hormone, cholecystokinin. This makes the gall bladder contract to squirt out alkaline bile. It also nudges the pancreas to release lipase in its definitive hardcover edition: pancreatic lipase.

Sugars and amino acids dissolve and acquire their visas immediately, ready for absorption.

Digesting oil is tricky, and for a very obvious reason.

Oil and water don't mix and the gut is one vast ocean. Fats will keep bouncing about in the Jacuzzi, refusing dissolution, like grease on a kitchen towel. That calls for soap!

And the small intestine has a very handy detergent.

Bile.

When the insoluble triglyceride meets up with bile salts, it gets emulsified.

The emulsified triglyceride is now easily broken down.

This takes care of more than 90 per cent of the fat.

The products of digestion, fatty acids, have short or long chains, depending on the number of carbon atoms. Short-chain fatty acids are absorbed immediately by the velvety villi in the intestinal lining. They pass directly into the capillaries and cruise in the bloodstream for a short trip to the liver where fatty acids are put to work immediately and converted into energy.

But there is still a large fraction of processed fats awaiting absorption. These are long-chained, too large to be mopped up by the villi's luxurious Turkish towel.

There are other fats too, besides the products of triglyceride breakdown. These are phospholipids, and—ah yes, the arch-villain in all body stories—CHOLESTEROL.

All these waiting lipids are helped into the cells of the intestinal lining (enterocytes) by a number of transfer proteins.

When the meal has been very oily, and there are a lot of lipids lined up, these proteins hurry them into the intestinal cells.

Once inside the enterocyte, these fragmented lipids are shipped off to the factory: the endoplasmic reticulum or ER. Here they are reassembled into triglycerides again. Unlike the oil in the biryani which existed only for pleasure, these newbie triglycerides are quickly equipped for a very long voyage. They acquire a coating of proteins and become large lipoprotein particles called *chylomicrons*. After further education, these chylomicrons, bulging with triglycerides, gather at the base of the enterocyte, ready to embark. Some stay back, as oil droplets in the enterocyte. These are insurance against starvation, when they will be pushed out into the circulation to be used for energy. This can also happen between meals. Does that act as a brake on the next meal? It's a thought.

The chylomicrons, those that get shipped out, are like the unwieldy galleons on which sixteenth-century adventurers explored the world.

Besides the blob of oil at its heart, a chylomicron also has fat-soluble vitamins, cholesterol esters, free cholesterol, phospholipids, and a very large protein shell called apolipoprotein. Which is to say, it is grease in every possible avatar.

Exiting chylomicrons glide into the lymphatic network around the enterocytes and paddle their way upstream out of the abdominal cavity. They do this inside the thoracic duct which ends in the large subclavian vein at the base of the neck. Here the lymphatic pipeline tips its load of grease into the bloodstream. The chylomicrons, bulging with oil, now race through the circulation.

The walls of the capillaries have cells that produce yet another edition of lipase, a festschrift this one, meant for keeps. Its job is to crack the lipoprotein, and so it is called lipoprotein lipase. Its release is controlled by the hormone insulin.

When chylomicrons flood the capillaries in adipose tissue, the adipocyte wakes up.

Insulin gets lipoprotein lipase going to crack the chylomicron into fatty acids, and encourages these fatty acids to enter the adipocyte.

What happens next?

Drumroll, please.

This is the point where a number of small, critical changes might lead up to the Big O.

The adipocyte relies on a number of signals to decide whether to store these fatty acids or to break down its existing store and ship it out.

Insulin stimulates lipoprotein lipase and encourages the adipocyte to form more triglycerides and enlarge its store of fat.

Opposing hormones, glucagon and adrenaline, counter this effect. Under their influence the fat inside the adipocyte breaks down into free fatty acids and glycerol.

Normally, as a meal is being digested, insulin has the upper hand. This means no free fatty acids are released into the blood from adipose tissue, and the adipocytes mop up fatty acids from those overburdened chylomicrons.

Meanwhile, insulin continues its good work by making the liver synthesize triglycerides from different sources, and float them out as Very Low Density Lipoprotein particles. These are eagerly accepted by the adipocyte, broken down, and added to its store of fat.

This assures two things:

- There's enough dietary fat to provide ready fuel for most of the body's cells.
- The excess is neatly packaged away in adipose tissue, to be mobilized as an energy source in lean times.

This is the perfectly rational dialogue between fat on the plate and the fat in the body.

Efficient, harmonic, sentient, it is practically a love song. It is, in fact, the oldest love song on the planet.

Rice Stories

Given the choice of one survival food, what would you choose?

'Rice!'

Every Indian has a rice story, and this is mine.

1967

That summer, there was a thunderstorm. The sky had lowered all afternoon, great rolling billows of soft grey. I sat on the garden steps watching the scurrying birds blown off course righting themselves hurriedly, bowled along by the wind that did not, yet, mean them harm.

The light changed abruptly, pale gold turning subtly and dangerously blue, before the first flash ripped the sky.

I had my eyes shut tight, waiting for thunder. It was still far off, clearing its throat somewhere.

I had promised myself I wouldn't open my eyes till I heard the first really loud rumble. When it came, it sounded as if someone was dragging heavy furniture above all those clouds. Disappointed, I opened my eyes.

It had turned dark. Then a spear of lightning shot overhead and thunder crashed and rumbled and drummed loud enough to console me.

Rain came, hot and slow, like tears.

All this I remember because, as I tasted the first raindrop on my tongue, I saw her.

She was crouched just beyond our fence of jungle-jalebi, shivering, hugging herself. She was dressed in over-sized bloomers, and nothing else.

The torrent broke and rain lashed with malice.

I cleared the garden in two leaps and pulled her in through a gap in the hedge. We huddled silently in the verandah, watching the rain.

When the rain stopped, she was gone.

She came every afternoon, and would stand waiting beyond the hedge till I pulled her in.

When I had known her a week, I asked her name.

'Balloon.'

That couldn't be true!

'Belu?'

'No. Balloon. But you can call me Belu, if you like.'

'Which do you like?'

'I like Belu.'

So Belu she became.

Her brothers had named her Balloon in jest, but neither Belu, nor I, thought that funny.

We didn't talk much.

We were friends because of Belu's game.

She set about it the moment she entered our garden.

She would scoop up a tuffet of soil from one of the flowerbeds and sit cross-legged on the grass. The crumbly clay turned smooth as chocolate in her coaxing palms.

I watched breathlessly at what emerged: exquisitely modelled figurines.

They were always the same. Pugilistic men, dainty broad-hipped ladies with conical breasts.

Belu was especially good with the women. She did their faces. Moulded ringlets over their foreheads. When they were nearly dry, she would find a tiny twig and with precise deliberation drill a crater atop each breast, and one in the midline precisely above the waistband of the pleated skirt.

Belu worked fast, never had much time to talk, and anyway, her fingers were nimbler than her tongue.

She worked as a maid in four houses, beginning at dawn.

Come evening, she returned to make chapattis in each of those houses, and in between, she had to cook for her own family.

She was friends with me because I sat silently watching while she made her clay people.

She ignored them the moment they were done. I had a shoebox full of them by now.

I gave her a dress of mine in exchange. She was pleased.

But the next day she again turned up in those ragged bloomers.

'Won't you wear the dress?' I asked.

For answer, she slapped her flat chest. 'Still some time for that.'

As I said, we didn't talk much.

I was afraid to ask, ashamed to tell. I knew that our hour together was purchased every time by my silence.

So it startled me when, one afternoon at the hedge, she said, 'I can't come in, I have to be home early, but you can come with me if you like.'

I scrambled out eagerly before she could change her mind.

She plodded on, disowning me.

I knew she lived beyond the ring of huts that fringed the horizon.

In those days, despite its proximity to the airport, Dum Dum was still surprisingly rural. You could stumble on a brake of trees behind a hoarding and find them clustered around a pukur, a stagnant pond choked with green scum. Sometimes there were hyacinths, delicate frills of blue and purple that wilted at first breath.

Belu led me past one such pukur, up an incline where pigs rooted about in the marsh. Then we were there, at her house, walking up the hard beaten steps to the porch.

It was the most exciting place I had seen.

The mud floor swabbed with gobar was scrupulously

clean. There was a pot of tulsi, another of periwinkle. A cat sunned itself on the ledge. On a clothesline hung the signature red gamcha of a Bengali household.

There was nobody at home.

Belu threw me a look and after that, ignored me.

I watched greedily, afraid it would all vanish if I blinked.

A large clay pot bubbled sulkily on a choolah in a corner of the porch. Belu squatted next to it and began stirring it with a wooden ladle. A blue haze of aromatic steam drew me closer.

'Rice.'

There was rice, somewhere, deep in the pot, but the milky froth that swelled and ebbed was a clear kanji.

I had never smelt anything as delicious before.

Belu stirred the pot and a few dark chunks came floating up.

'We have a banana today,' she said proudly. 'And a brinjal. That's for Baba.'

She explained her brothers would be coming in for lunch and she would have hers now.

She went into the dark interior of the hut, leaving me to watch the pot.

She returned with a brass bowl that shone like gold. Into it she ladled kanji—once, and then with hesitation, a second time. It barely covered the bottom of the bowl.

We squatted on either side, faces laved in steam.

Belu cupped her hands around the bowl and held it out to me to sip. Then with an impatient cluck, drew it back, blew on it, swirled it around, tested it with the tip of her little finger and offered it to me again.

In the clear broth, tiny flecks of rice floated like jasmine.

I took it from her and sipped.

All the flavours in the world revealed themselves in that mouthful.

It was sharp with salt and silky with the subtle sweetness

of starch. The rice melted on my tongue like dew. I raised my eyes to meet her anxious gaze.

As she took the bowl from me, I saw her smile for the first time.

When she had drained the bowl and licked it clean, her brothers turned up, big noisy lads who spurned me. The older one helped himself from the pot.

'Leave the banana for Baba,' Belu barked sharply.

The boy fished out the chunk from his bowl and slipped it back into the pot. He filled his bowl to the brim and took himself away from my contaminating gaze to eat.

Belu stirred the pot and added more water.

The younger brother waited for Belu to fill his bowl. She dropped in a chunk of brinjal and ladled some rice into the kanji. The boy hesitated.

'I've eaten. Go finish before Baba turns up,' Belu said roughly.

Round and red and shiny through the steam, she looked very like her name.

After the boys left, Belu scoured the bowl and spread a straw mat on the floor before she went back to stirring the pot, waiting for her father.

Baba was some time coming up the path, a little heavy with toddy. He stopped at the steps to take a leak. I looked away, embarrassed.

'*Ki Khokhi*?' he roared as he came up.

I crept into the shadows, hoping he wouldn't notice me.

He didn't.

He sat down on the mat and waited to be served.

Belu filled the bowl. This time it was filled with rice.

After she had set it down, almost shyly, she crowned the fluffy mound with a chunk of banana.

Baba made an appreciative sound and set to.

Belu fanned him with a palm leaf.

When the bowl was half-empty, she filled it again. There were more vegetables.

On the floor next to him, she served a small hillock of salt. He dipped the vegetables in salt delicately, one by one.

When he was done, he pushed the bowl away pettishly, and asked, 'Is that all then? How is a man to fill his stomach on this morsel?'

Belu added a ladle of kanji unwillingly.

He splashed it on the wall and stalked out in a rage.

I was trembling with fury and dread.

I didn't dare to look at Belu's rigid back as she added more water and stirred the pot again.

After a while I couldn't bear it, and went up to her.

There was very little left in the pot, just a thin grey scum of starch in the swirling water. Belu took out the ladle and covered the pot.

'It will be done by the time mother comes in,' she said. 'Let's go, or I'll be late.'

2017

On 28 September, ten-year-old Santoshi Kumari died asking for a mouthful of rice. She had eaten nothing for eight days.

In Karimati, Jharkhand, households lost their ration cards to a new Government Rule: Ration cards not linked to an Aadhar Number by 5 April 2017 were all defunct.

The Aadhaar Scheme* is presently under review by the Supreme Court. In principle, it is a flagrant violation of the citizen's right to privacy. In practice, it is a head count

*The Hindi word *Aadhaar* means 'foundation' or 'basis.' The *Aadhaar Number* is a twelve-digit random number issued by the UIDAI (Unique Identification Authority of India) to the residents of India after satisfying the verification process which includes demographic (Name, date of birth (verified) or age (declared), gender, address, mobile number (optional) and email ID (optional)) and biometric (ten fingerprints, two iris scans, and facial photograph) information.

brutally reminiscent of Nazi Germany. In Digital India, it is one more opportunity for corruption and oppression.

Even before the Central government order came into force, there were reports of ration shops refusing to honour ration cards not linked with Aadhaar.

The irony is that Santoshi's mother, Koyli Devi, did possess an Aadhaar card. It just wasn't linked with her ration card. Why? The online portal wasn't working or there was no internet connectivity.

Whatever the reason, the horrific truth cannot be denied. The family starved for eight days, and nobody helped.

Everyone knew they were starving, Koyli Devi begged her neighbours for food. 'If there are any leftovers, sure,' they assured her.

There never were any leftovers.

Is it so difficult to share a meal?

In our India today, it is.

Nothing has become so alien to us as greeting a neighbour, or sharing a meal with a stranger.

I don't have to go to Karimati to meet Santoshi's family. They are all around me on the streets of India's richest metropolis. But they are invisible.

Santoshi's school had closed for Durga Puja, else she would have had, at least, the school lunch every day.

Koyli Devi and her older daughter earned a pittance by cutting grass. It was all the income their family had.

While these facts are in the public domain, we are excluded from the private domain of Santoshi's experience.

Since this story broke in early October, I have been haunted by one question: *Through those eight days of total starvation, what did Santoshi feel?*

Today everyone knows Santoshi. Her face stares at us thoughtfully. There is a calm defiance in her eyes. Yes, in a minute she will have to humour the toddler at her hip, return to being big sister or little mother. But in this blink of time, she looks her question at the world.

On a good day, Santoshi perhaps ate about one-third of her energy requirement of 1,600 calories. Reports about the prevalent diet in Santoshi's neighbourhood suggest that children there have long been victims of protein-calorie malnutrition. Hunger is appeased with watery meals of rice kanji.

This would have been Santoshi's 'normal'.

Within her family, food would be apportioned hierarchically: with Santoshi at the end of the line. This too was 'normal'.

The change that killed Santoshi was not unforeseen. Her body had assembled a compensatory metabolism through a childhood of deprivation. But what she experienced in the last week of life was devastatingly sudden. Having very little to eat was replaced by having *nothing* to eat.

There was no rice left. No potatoes. No flour.

When food ran out, they were hungry, perhaps she most of all.

Her mother sent her out to the neighbours to borrow food. They shooed her away. She dawdled outside, dreading a return home empty-handed.

The elders drowsed. The little ones howled.

Santoshi no longer felt hungry, just angry.

She lay on her stomach, thinking.

They tried to wake her, but she wanted to be left alone. Light hurt her eyes.

She staggered out to the gutter to relieve herself. That was yesterday.

Her mother fussed, worried that Santoshi was running a fever.

Perhaps she was, Santoshi was past caring. She was just cold.

Her mother brought her a drink of hot water. It roused her enough to sit up.

In a little while she curled up again.

'My head hurts,' she told her mother. 'I feel faint.'

'Get on your feet,' her mother implored. 'I'll help you walk about a little.'

Santoshi's knees buckled and she slipped to the floor, dragging her mother with her.

The story now becomes discordant.

In the first version, Koyli Devi took Santoshi to the doctor after the child blacked out.

The doctor's prescription was terse. 'Feed her a meal.'

'What about medicine?'

'All she needs is food.'

This version isn't very convincing. Unlikely that a household without coin for food will have the resource to consult a doctor.

The second version says that Koyli Devi did not take her daughter to the doctor.

The third version (the Government's version) says that Santoshi was taken to a doctor who diagnosed malaria. It was malaria, not starvation, that killed her.

More versions will swirl around in this simoom of surmise, dust in our eyes, to keep us from seeing what it was like for Santoshi, now in her eighth, and final, day of starvation.

The effort of speaking or moving is insurmountable. She is cold all the time. Curled up against the wall, she answers her mother's touch with just one word, 'Bhaat.'

It is her last word before she slips imperceptibly from drowsiness into coma into death.

It is the only word Koyli Devi recalls.

The voice of a dying child, begging for a morsel of rice.

To Belu and to Santoshi, fifty years apart in time, the perfect meal meant a mouthful of rice.

What does it mean to you?

The Body Politic

We are divided by language. We Indians are, by necessity polyglot, macaronic. And, the great equalizer, English, mothers every subcontinental inflection and idiom. We have evolved (we hope) from the scorn we had fifty years ago towards each other's language. We aren't so deaf any more. We understand now that our deafness was mere ignorance. We haven't yet forsworn the malice of that ignorance. There are private slurs, of course, but also very public ones which caricature and denigrate 'the other'. Such injuries are never forgotten, the insult is even harder to forgive. Our sullen rage inspissates into a wall of exclusivity, isolation, alienation, and hate.

The body, too, is polyglot. Its various members speak variously, and are hard put to comprehend each other.

The mutiny of body parts has been exploited as metaphor for the body politic in every culture through the ages, perhaps never so pithily as in the opening scene of Shakespeare's *Coriolanus*.

There was a time when all the body's members
Rebell'd against the belly, thus accused it:
That only like a gulf it did remain
I' the midst o' the body, idle and unactive,
Still cupboarding the viand, never bearing
Like labour with the rest, where the other instruments
Did see and hear, devise, instruct, walk, feel,
And, mutually participate, did minister

Unto the appetite and affection common
Of the whole body.

In obesity, the body is on the verge of mutiny; Metabolic Syndrome and diabetes are just around the corner. It is a cogent moment to address a reproach to the belly:

The kingly-crowned head, the vigilant eye,
The counsellor heart, the arm our soldier,
Our steed the leg, the tongue our trumpeter.
With other muniments and petty helps
In this our fabric, if that they—

Should by the cormorant belly be restrain'd,
Who is the sink o' the body,—

The belly answers:

'True is it, my incorporate friends,' quoth he,
'That I receive the general food at first,
Which you do live upon; and fit it is,
Because I am the store-house and the shop
Of the whole body: but, if you do remember,
I send it through the rivers of your blood,
Even to the court, the heart, to the seat o' the brain;
And, through the cranks and offices of man,
The strongest nerves and small inferior veins
From me receive that natural competency
Whereby they live:

Every body part has a point of view and deserves a hearing before the cormorant belly caps the discussion.

As is only natural, we begin, with 'the kingly crowned head'—the brain.

The Brain's Story

We saw earlier how we grew ourselves a brain. We saw, too, that the brain calls the shots about what we eat.

But, *how does the brain eat?*

Wrapped in the Blood-Brain-Barrier (B-B-B), in all its awful majesty, the brain is a daunting customer to feed. It isn't a simple matter of shovelling glucose across the capillary lining, we know the cell wall will unzip with alacrity and snatch lunch.

The brain does not stand for such familiarity, even though, usually, there's just one dish on the menu, glucose. Yes, if you're fasting, or you're diabetic, the brain will accept ketones as well.

Let us look at the healthy brain on a good day.

Cells called astrocytes make up most of the brain's supporting tissue. Astrocytes are in close contact with endothelial cells in the walls of brain capillaries. Astrocytes and endothelial cells express various types of Glucose Transporters (GLUTs) that permit the entry of glucose into the cell. They alter the permeability of the Blood-Brain-Barrier to the glucose molecule. GLUT-1 is expressed in the cells of the B-B-B and more strongly in astrocytes. GLUT-1 is only partially sensitive to insulin.* GLUT 3 is expressed strongly in neurons, and is insulin sensitive.

For years the brain was dismissed as 'insulin-insensitive'. A monster that grabbed every passing molecule of glucose without giving a damn about the body's metabolic status, as it stayed focussed on its own.

Insulin receptors are widely distributed in the brain. Insulin crosses the B-B-B and is also present in Cerebro-Spinal Fluid (CSF). While most of the glucose uptake by the brain is insulin-independent, a fraction is still insulin sensitive.

The regional differences in insulin sensitivity might be a protective mechanism. In starvation (low circulating

---

*GLUT-1 deficiency in astrocytes has been seen in degenerative illnesses like Alzheimer's Disease.

glucose states), this diverts glucose to the parts of the brain necessary for survival, like the brainstem. This happens even by denying glucose to the 'thinking brain'.

The brain has two complementary ways of dealing with glucose.

Neurons convert glucose oxidatively: each molecule of glucose yields thirty-eight molecules of Adenosine Tri-Pphosphate (ATP) as energy.

Astrocytes opt for a different path, a glycolytic one, where glucose is changed into lactate and pyruvate. These two end molecules are then transferred onto neurons where they are converted into ATP.

Astrocytes, as their name suggests, look like stars. These pretty cells were described more than a century ago, but only now are we learning of their role in the brain's metabolism. Astrocytes literally straddle the blood-brain divide. All the brain's capillaries are roofed with astrocyte 'end-feet'. These are extensions from the astrocyte cell body. The astrocyte has other extensions that synapse with surrounding cells.

The brain can utilize lactate directly from the plasma. After vigorous exercise, when blood lactate levels rise, the brain can use it for as much as 20 per cent of its energy needs. The lactate from astrocytes is used particularly to establish long-term memory.

This allows the brain some latitude in its choice of nutrients. The brain is a big eater. It takes up 25 per cent of the day's quota of calories. This is largely because we raced ahead of chimpanzees in cognition. As the neocortex increased in size, we got the ability to think and to use language, and a staggering number of new neurons were added.

We have an estimated 16 billion neurons. Non-human primates have less than half that number.

The brain feeds at the expense of the rest of the body. This finding dates back to 1921 when researcher Marie Krieger described that in starvation, while other body organs lost 40 per cent weight, the brain weight remained unaffected.

The brain has two broad categories of performers: *excitatory neurons* which use the chemical glutamate and *inhibitory neurons* which use GABA (Gamma-AminoButyric Acid). When ATP levels fall, excitatory neurons fire and release glutamate. Glutamate renders the astrocytes more absorptive. Glucose levels in CSF also rise. The Hypothalamic-Pitutary-Adrenal Axis and the sympathetic nervous system are activated. We register hunger, and are compelled to imbibe a good whack of carbohydrates. So far, so clear.

Now for the surprise.

We would expect a sugar-loaded treat to be followed by an immediate rebuke—a rise in circulating insulin.

This does not happen.

The stressed brain actually suppresses the release of insulin. As a consequence, other body tissues which require insulin for glucose entry and utilization, starve, while the brain gluts on sugar for its own needs.

This Selfish Brain Theory was propounded in 1998 by Achim Peters. Since then, it has been extended to explain feeding, satiation, and, yes, obesity.

Experimentally, subjects under stress experience 'neuroglycopenia': sweating, tremors, anxiety and hunger—even though their blood sugar levels are normal. Led to a generous buffet, they eagerly feed on carbohydrate foods (without discriminating between sweet and non-sweet)—and soon feel better.

If they are fed salads instead and denied a hit of carbohydrate, they continue to feel uncomfortable for a long period after the stress. This suggests the brain seeks out carbohydrates to meet its demands under stress. As the brain gates insulin, other tissues don't get a snack.

This experiment is common experience with most of us. We are pretty familiar with this, aren't we? We call it 'comfort eating'.

According to the Selfish Brain Theory, this mechanism is altered in obesity. Under stress, we do glut on carbohydrate, but the brain is not prioritized and energy excess accumulates across all tissues, leading to fat deposition and weight gain.

The brain views our need for food like a sensible cook. It offers us a plain fare menu and a festive one.

Plain fare keeps life going. The posh term for this is *homeostasis*. Biochemically, this means a stable blood sugar and normal serum lipids. Structurally, it means body weight within acceptable limits, no excessive fat deposits, and a decent amount of lean body mass.

Examine this family-style restaurant in the brain:

The kitchen is the Hypothalamus. For nearly a century, it has been the focus of avid research, but we're still on the threshold of understanding. Until a few years ago, three principal stations in the hypothalamus were assigned different functions, but now we have a newer, more plastic, model that explains how it works.

Think of it as a kitchen located between the dining room and the pantry. From the dining room comes information about the customer, and the world outside. From the pantry derives the inside view of ingredients. The chef has to match the two, and accordingly deliver either plain fare or fine dining.

In the brain, the hypothalamus is located between the brainstem and the cortico-limbic system.

The brainstem gets information from rest of the body through the vagus and from hormones in circulation; it also sends back directives through these messengers. It decides how much we eat.

The cortico-limbic system is a catch-all term for the

network between the 'newer' thinking and discriminating part of the brain and the 'older' impulsive and emotional pleasure seeking part. This network discerns 'food clues' in our perception of the outside world. The emotions they evoke are linked to memory and experience, and will translate into pleasure or aversion.

The hypothalamus then integrates all this information, and settles on a menu that pleases and satisfies—but it must also maintains metabolic balance.

How does it pull off this feat even-handedly?

Very secretly.

We're never aware of what is happening till we respond to it.

Before we consider how the hypothalamus processes energy intake, let us see how the body spends energy.

How much energy do we need?

Energy expenditure = Energy for basal metabolic processes + Energy expended in physical activity + 'Food thermogenesis'—burning calories to provide warmth, carried out by brown fat.

When energy intake and energy expenditure are equalized (Energy Homeostasis), we maintain an acceptable body weight.

It is this equation we must examine in any discussion of obesity.

For long it was believed that there is a fixed 'set point' for body weight as a result of efficient homeostasis. This means that any divergence from this set point due to eating too much or too little, or eating the wrong stuff, will revert to the expected body weight once you eat right.

This is a neat fairy-tale scenario, cute, but not believable.

Look around you, and you'll agree.

If I stop bingeing on pastry and farsan and go back to 'normal home food', will my waist return to its former slender self?

Not bloody likely, as every overweight reader knows, to his or her grief.

This is the reason why most 'diets' fail.

The brain has simply reset its 'set point'. Or more correctly, *there is no set point*, just a sneakily sliding one.

The Lateral Hypothalamic Area (LHA) has long been regarded as the 'feeding centre'. It releases orexins and gets you ravenous. But this is too naïve. The LHA is too well connected with other parts of the brain, and other parts of the hypothalamus as well, to act with such savage greed. It also registers rewards of pleasure and satiety. The connections it makes with the adjacent Arcuate Nucleus may inhibit the release of anorexins, and so get you interested in lunch. Its connections with the brainstem compel second helpings, and make you linger rather longer than usual at the dining table.

The LHA today seems a sophisticated decision-maker. It makes the decision to feed based on both nutritional and emotional needs relayed to it from the body's internal milieu as well as external stimuli. It also decides satiety.

Remember leptin, the hormone secreted by the adipocyte?

There are Leptin Receptor Neurons in the LHA which project on neurons that release orexin, suggesting that leptin may directly control greed.

The adjacent Arcuate Nucleus has AgRP* neurons which stimulate feeding. Leptin inhibits them. So does insulin. Ghrelin, the greed hormone from the stomach, stimulates them.

---

*Agouti-related protein, AgRP, is a signaling molecule identified in 1997. The agouti is a Central and South American rodent related to the guinea pig. Agouti also refers to grizzly fur, where each hair has alternate dark and light bands.

The Arcuate Nucleus also has POMC* neurons—these inhibit feeding. Leptin stimulates them into releasing anorexins. Ghrelin inhibits them.

What is the brain's response to the stress of low blood sugar?

Imagine the discomfort you feel when you skip a meal. Hunger, of course, but you're forced to ignore that—there is no food at hand. You feel tired. Your head aches. You resent present company and lash out at the least provocation. You feel light-headed, and perhaps black out. But gradually, though the prospect of a meal remains very distant, you begin to recover. You are still tired, but in better humour. That headache has let up. You get on with the day, but take it slow, with your feet up.

What exactly has the brain been up to?

It has pressed the alarm button: stopped insulin secretion, and upped all the opposing adrenergic hormones by activating the Hypothalamic-Pituitary-Adrenal axis.

It is the Selfish Mode in full operation. The brain keeps going on the glucose it has stolen from your muscles.

This is also the picture in Metabolic Syndrome and obesity—and surprise, surprise, in diabetes when the blood sugar levels are high.

Why should completely different scenarios provoke the same response?

The brain seems to respond to signals of both immediate energy status (blood sugar) as well as long-term energy status (leptin signalling).

In Metabolic Syndrome, obesity and diabetes, the levels of circulating leptin are high but the brain ignores this signal. It exhibits Leptin Resistance.

*Pro-opiomelanocortin (POMC) is a polypeptide synthesized in the pituitary gland. It is necessary to produce hormones.

Leptin Receptors are everywhere—in the brain, and all over the rest of the body. Judging from their ubiquity, it certainly appears as if the adipocyte controls the narrative, since it is the only source of leptin.

Leptin is the body's most reliable bulletin of energy status. But only in the healthy, insulin-effective, acceptable-BMI body

Leptin loses credibility as you begin to pile on fat. Within the spectrum of obesity, Metabolic Syndrome and diabetes, leptin is just just fake news.

It cheerily announces 'All's well and booming, and it's time to lay off the fats and sugars!' But the body's isn't listening. More particularly, the brain isn't listening.

Naturally, Leptin Resistance has been, for some time, the focus of much agonized research. What have we gleaned about it?

Leptin and insulin act together. They also fail together. So the two hormones are often studied in tandem.

Endoplasmic Reticulum (ER) Stress has been identified as the leading cause of both leptin and insulin resistance.

The ER is a cell organelle which performs quality control on the folding of proteins synthesized in the cell. If a protein is misfolded, it is junked, and it accumulates in the ER causing ER Stress. To overcome this, the Unfolded Protein Response is activated to clear up the mess.

ER Stress is the common denominator in metabolic, neurodegenerative and neoplastic disease.

Recently, the excessive intake of saturated fats has been shown to increase ER Stress.

Experimentally, ER Stress leads to both insulin and leptin resistance.

Two molecules have been identified as causing leptin and insulin resistance: Suppressor of Cytokine Signalling 3 (SOCS3), and protein tyrosine phosphatase 1B (PTP1B).

It is clear that insulin and leptin act not just in tandem, they act synergistically on the hypothalamus. One theory postulates that high levels of circulating fat prevent the entry of leptin through the B-B-B. But there is growing evidence for a second theory: hypothalamic inflammation.

Oh yes, that's possible. For a while now, both 'involuntary' weight loss (without obvious cause) and obesity have been related to inflammatory changes in the hypothalamus. In obesity we know there is peripheral inflammation—but it may have been preceded by inflammation in the hypothalamus.

Observations in laboratory animals—rats, mice, non-human primates—show that within 48–72 hours of being fed a high fat diet, the hypothalamus reacts with glial over-activity and production of cytokines, chemical attractants that get inflammatory cells revved up. This initial response occurs way ahead of any change in adipose depots. As yet, this response is protective, the changes being restricted to the glial cells only. But if the high-fat diet is continued, inflammation becomes established, markers show up in the neurons themselves, suggesting that actual injury has occurred.

Why does that happen?

Clearly, it is related to the nutritional overload. Short-chain fatty acids have been implicated, and it is likely that the inflammation is leptin mediated. It is also interesting that this 'established inflammation' is reversible if the high-fat diet is stopped and healthier feeds substituted.

Chemokines released by glial cells in the inflamed hypothalamus may be the key to altering the balance between anorexigenic and orexigenic chemicals, and tipping the balance in favour of obesity.

In this narrative, the brain accepts responsibility for tweaking the feeding-satiety cycle, but that only came about because of an overload of nutrients. So the cormorant stomach stays accused.

The brain's 'I told you so' is based on the 'strongest nerves' that Shakespeare alluded to in the stomach's discourse. Between the stomach and the brain there is a very strong nerve that would have delighted Shakespeare.

The Vagus

I am that merry wanderer of the night.

—*A Midsummer Night's Dream;*
Act 2, Scene 1

Imagine a Puck within your body, a shrewd and knavish sprite, not really malicious, but up to all sorts of tricks that can puzzle and embarrass you. People with 'indigestion' will readily confirm that it is probable, not just possible. Certainly, there is something puckish about the tummy.

Whether Shakespeare knew of it or not, the culprit is a merry wanderer. And has been so named since 1856. Earlier, when it was named at all, it was called the pneumo-gastric nerve. Now, we call it vagus, the wanderer.

It begins its journey from the brain, it is designated tenth among the twelve cranial nerves.

With a parting handshake with its old friend the ninth nerve, it exits the skull in exalted company, the major blood vessels of the brain. This gets it a bit swollen, and it gives the eleventh nerve the barest nod, and it seems all set to sail sedately down the neck ignoring the lowlife. But, like all wanderers, it is curious as hell. So it sends off branches to the ear and the skin and chats up the seventh and ninth nerves while reeling in all the gossip from the back of the throat. Our awaara whistles as he wanders into the vocal cords. The next time you say something truly awful, blame it on the vagus.

All that gossip counts for something, and the vagus faithfully reports back to HQ. Like European travellers of an earlier age trawling the mysterious East, the vagus is not so much tramp as spy. It lacks Chaplin's honour, and it always tells.

It is also something of a snob, is our vagus. After that bit of slumming, it pats down its whiskers and keeps close to royalty—the magnificent blood vessels—as it swaggers into the chest. Although, true to its sneaky nature, it has sent ahead an exploratory branch all the way to the heart.

Here it is then, sliding down behind the heart, along the lungs. A shirker as ever, it slips slyly behind the throbbing machinery of the chest and snuggles up against the oesophagus as it begins the most exciting part of its travels. All this while, it stays in touch with all its new cronies and keeps the brain posted on every little peccadillo above the diaphragm.

It really comes out of the closet in the abdomen and turns respectable, forming the right and left gastric nerves and the celiac nerve, networking with everything that is anything in the abdominal cavity. The stomach and the intestines are totally in thrall to the vagus, as are the liver, spleen, pancreas and kidneys.

With its newfound respectability it stays clear of the pelvis, leaving the dirty work to lowlife from the spinal cord. It still gets all the gossip!

The vagus could well boast like Puck, 'I jest to Oberon and make him smile.'

Shakespeare's Oberon is very like our brain. He has spies everywhere. He is greedy and very acquisitive, and not easily shamed. Like his Greek original, Zeus, he is a punishing bully, and Puck's mischief can have unintended consequences. See now how our Puck's jests to his Oberon lead up to obesity.

Like any hobo, the vagus takes orders very unwillingly. It is much better at picking up and relaying information—and what a lot of news that is!

Towards the stomach, it is a rude mechanical. All it wants to know about the stomach is: just how full is it?

But lower down the intestine, the vagus displays chemical intelligence.

Together, the mechanicals and the chemical smarts establish a neat system of—STOPPING THE MEAL.

Satiation—the strong signal which makes us stop eating is a truly Puckish prank.

This is how it works. As the stomach fills, the elastic muscle wall stretches to accommodate food, the vagus telegraphs this to the brain which starts off its anorexins, and before I know it, I'm refusing a second helping of that delectable biryani.

But it isn't that easy.

When the stomach was empty, special cells in the lining squeezed out a lot of ghrelin, the only orexin the gut manufactures. When the vagus gets iffy about the distending stomach, ghrelin opposes it. If ghrelin wins, I can manage just a little bit more of the biryani.

Like the tramp that it is, the vagus is not discriminating. It does equal justice to carbohydrate, protein or fat—or even for that matter, water. It only registers stomach stretch.

The chemical intelligence is more sophisticate. The vagus doesn't dangle its feet in the mess within the intestines. It steps prettily about the clever cells in the intestinal lining, the entero-endocrine cells that sense different nutrients swirling about in the jacuzzi. These cells secrete hormones in response to the menu. For instance, the fats and proteins in biryani are picked up immediately by cells which secrete cholecystokinin (CCK). This, we've known for years, makes the gall bladder contract to release bile and aid in the digestion of fats—but this happens a little later.

The immediate action of CCK is to inform the vagus that there is plenty of fat in the lunch. The vagus relays this to the brain which issues an embargo instantly, and I leave the table without clearing my plate. And that's just CCK. There are many more hormones (thirty-two and counting) which work in the same manner. This makes the vagus a regular buzzkill just when I was getting ready to really pig out.

As if this weren't enough, vagal fibres in the liver sense the arrival of a fresh load of nutrients in the portal vein, and hasten this information to the brain which clamps down severely on the meal.

The vagus has its own brand of justice. If I've been hungry too long, if I'm low on energy, the vagus holds back its strictures and I can eat a little more.

The vagus is more than a killjoy that ends the meal. It has important things to do in digesting and absorbing what I've eaten. And for these actions, it transmits orders from the brain. It is this part of the vagus' profile that surgeons my age are all too familiar with.

When I was a surgical resident thirty years ago, the commonest operation done every week was listed as 'Vagotomy G-J'. It was used to treat peptic ulcer.

Never mind that patients recovered from surgery only to develop fresh ulcers.

Never mind that they also developed a slew of new problems.

That operation, happily, is long abandoned, and only to be recalled with a shudder.

I mention it here because it focussed on a very important function of the vagus nerve: its action on the parietal cells of the stomach lining which increase their secretion of acid. It was thought that severing the vagus nerve would alleviate high stomach acidity and allow the ulcer a chance to heal—which it did.

Stomach acid is essential for normal digestion. Without vagal activity, this would not be maintained at optimum. The muscle at the stomach outlet, the pylorus, forms a 'sphincter'—a ring that constricts to seal off contents and opens up only to empty the stomach. The vagus constricts this outlet, retains stomach contents, so they can be churned and doused in acid to optimize its action.

The Migrating Motor Complex is a four-phased cycle of intestinal movement observed during fasting. It begins in the lower stomach or in the duodenum, and is responsible for preparing the intestine mechanically and chemically for the arrival of food. The vagus starts this cycle of movement and ensures that it is sustained by increasing the output of gastro-intestinal hormones like ghrelin and motilin.

With so much for the vagus to do, any number of things could go wrong affecting satiation, digestion and absorption.

At first glance it seems as though the vagus has tight control over satiation and therefore helps me to stop eating—but it has little or no role to play in long-term metabolic balance.

In obesity, vagal sensitivity to signals from intestinal hormones like CCK are dampened. This has been demonstrated experimentally in rats fed a high-fat diet.

The vagus also becomes quickly insensitive to leptin.

Both mechanisms contribute to over-eating!

In animals rendered obese experimentally, the vagus shows a blunted response to signals from the gut and addles information to the brain. This makes the animals glut.

Why does this happen?

Why does our merry wanderer become confused and stupid in obesity?

We have no answers yet.

Instead, there are plans to harness the vagus into performing therapeutically.

As we'll soon find out, this is tangential to the problem at hand.

And so, despite this strongest of nerves, it is still all about the stomach.

The Cormorant Stomach

> 'True is it, my incorporate friends,' quoth he,
> 'That I receive the general food at first,
> Which you do live upon; and fit it is,
> Because I am the store-house and the shop
> Of the whole body: but, if you do remember,
> I send it through the rivers of your blood,
> Even to the court, the heart, to the seat o' the brain;
> And, through the cranks and offices of man,
> The strongest nerves and small inferior veins
> From me receive that natural competency
> Whereby they live:
>
> —*Coriolanus*, Act 1, Scene 1

Shakespeare's Stomach makes a brave answer, even if it does take on responsibilities that, more properly, belong to the small intestine.

Still, its importance in obesity is a paradox. It is easily conceded in popular imagination, and more grudgingly, by science. Petuk, pet puja, thondi, and a dozen other such appellations in every Indian language, convey a common metaphor of greed. Science agrees quickly. Orexigenic ghrelin is the greedy hormone.

The stomach is perceived as a passive receptacle, even though it accomplishes many crucial things.

The small intestine seems much more worthy of respect as it bullies the stomach quite effectively with its orchestra of anorexigenic molecules.

Nearly a hundred years ago, confronted by an illness we didn't understand, it seemed perfectly logical to hack out a vital body part and throw it away.

At the beginning of the twentieth century, a very popular therapy for 'madness' was prefrontal lobotomy. It was pioneered by the Portuguese neurologist Antonio Egaz

Moniz who was awarded the Nobel in 1949. Lobotomy is, more correctly, *lobec*tomy, the ablation of neural tracts in the frontal lobes.

Moniz himself never did get his hands dirty, he merely influenced surgeons to perform the procedure.

It was popularized in the United States by Walter Freeman who developed the notorious technique by which the brain could be dug out in shreds with an ice-pick cleverly inserted into the angle of the eye. Freeman's technique did away with fussy details, like anaesthesia and asepsis. He did a messier job than the ancient Egyptians who removed the brains of their dead piecemeal through the nostril before mummifying them.

Freeman performed more than 3,000 surgeries, toured mental institutions across the continent, and left behind a trail of patients either dead or helplessly crippled.

We are at another Freeman moment now, only this time it isn't about the phantoms of the brain, but the very tangible and weighty problem of obesity.

The truth is, we don't yet know what the stomach does in obesity, and have long concluded it does nothing much at all.

Whenever human ignorance is unmasked, the reaction is predictable: violence. And we have been brutally violent with the stomach, cutting, stapling, banding, constricting and choking the life out of it in ham-fisted attempts to 'control' it, through procedures lumped together pretentiously as 'bariatric surgery'.*

The stomach is more than a tote that can be stuffed to capacity and then neatly tucked away beneath the ribs. Its

---

**Baros* is Greek for 'weight.' A *barometer* is an instrument to measure air pressure or weight. *Bariatric* was minted in 1965 by combining *baros*, 'weight' and *iatros*, 'healer' to describe medical treatment of the seriously overweight state—obesity.

geography is shaped by its function. The top (fundus) and the body make up 80 per cent of the secretory area of the stomach lining. The stomach secretes strong hydrochloric acid. This acid doesn't corrode the stomach wall because of a protective layer of mucus. Digestion in the stomach cannot begin without acid. This is the site of initial protein digestion, and acid activates the necessary enzyme. When acid secretion irritates the stomach lining, it sets off a familiar group of discomforts—acid peptic disease or dyspepsia.

Over the past two decades, Indians have been popping H_2 inhibitors, like Ranitidine, and proton pump inhibitors, like Omeprazole, by the ton. This has very definitely altered the delicate balance of the stomach milieu. We might soon be seeing the long-term consequences of such iatrogenic manipulation of stomach acidity in epidemic proportions—and it won't be pretty. In mice, the consequence, simply put, is stomach cancer.

The remaining 20 per cent of the stomach, the antrum, the exit to the duodenum, has a different secretion. This is the hormone gastrin.

Gastrin is secreted soon after food enters the stomach.

When stomach acid levels fall, gastrin secretion increases. Its job is to keep the stomach enzymes active and to relax the pyloric sphincter, the muscle that controls the stomach's exit.

In addition to these principal secretions, the stomach produces other molecules too:

- ''Intrinsic factor'—a substance needed to absorb dietary Vitamin B_{12}.
- Pepsinogen, that can be activated to digest proteins.
- And a number of neuroendocrine peptides.

The second major hormone secreted by the stomach is the greed hormone, ghrelin. This comes from the upper part of the stomach.

Ghrelin levels are inversely related to body weight. Most

obese people have low circulating ghrelin levels. But some do not.

We would expect ghrelin levels to fall after weight loss induced by bariatric surgery. This, too, is unpredictable. We know that ghrelin secretion is spurred by sympathetic activity and dampened by glucose. How do all these features add up to obesity?

The stomach also secretes a modest jot of leptin, but the major leptin contributor is adipose tissue. A third hormone, somatostatin, secreted by the stomach antrum, applies a powerful brake on all stomach functions. It reduces stomach secretions and reduces its motility too. Its overall effect is to slow down digestion.

Hormones from lower down the intestinal tract: CCK, secretin, GLP-1, GIP, (known collectively as entero-gastrones or incretin) work in concert to suppress acid secretion, so when the mush enters the duodenum, it is more easily rendered alkaline by bile.

The stomach is no couch potato. It is forever in a state of muscular activity, even between meals. The upper part of the stomach works towards storing and mixing food with gastric secretions. The lower part continues this mixing of food and directs its exit into the duodenum.

The muscular activity of the stomach at rest is its intrinsic tick, and originates from a pacemaker placed in middle of the antrum. This fasting activity (the Migrating Motor Complex) clears the stomach of undigested food, cleanses the lining, and prepares it for the next meal.

When we begin a meal, the pressure inside the stomach drops, the stomach wall distends, and we can gorge without discomfort until we're satiated.

The swallowed food is now thoroughly mixed with acid and the proteins in it are digested by the enzyme pepsin.

Meanwhile the pacemaker starts off more a vigorous

muscular movement—*peristalsis*. This is a crush-tear-pulverize session that makes teeth look like absolute kindergartners.

The stuff that exits the stomach bears no resemblance whatsoever to your gourmet lunch. Nonetheless, it has the consistency and texture any chef would be proud to call mousseline—smooth and silky, like a fine hollandaise. If detritus persists, an added nudge of muscle is all that's needed to decant it into the duodenum.

How soon does the stomach empty after a meal?

That depends on the meal.

Carbohydrates are quickly dispatched. Proteins take longer, and so do fats.

Hot foods move quicker, cold desserts sit it out.

The small intestine accepts small change only—4 calories per minute.

And then, above all, there is the unaccountable factor—your state of mind. When you're worried or sad, you simply don't feel hungry because the stomach is taking pause.

In most accounts, the stomach is seen as a rude mechanical, announcing satiation only when distended to bursting, while the small intestine has an elegant way of ending the meal well ahead of a burp.

Again, untrue.

Just examine the traditional menu of a feast in any part of the subcontinent, and you will notice the appetizers always include a bitter dish: the commonest ingredient is karela, followed by fenugreek (methi), neem, or orange peel.

The stomach lining has 'bitter receptors' that induce a rush of ghrelin.

In other words, the appetizer gets you hungry.

Soon after the first course, a broth either of meat (shorba) or daal (yusha, rasam) is usual. These are 'palate cleansers' meant to recharge the appetite. They do this not only because of their exquisite flavouring, but also because the peptones they contain are sensed immediately by the gastric mucosa which then responds with a surge of gastrin.

And, predictably, there is an evolutionary memory to this.

Bitter taste receptors are the most ubiquitous—not only are they in the mouth and throat, but also in large numbers in the stomach and small intestine. They always compel the secretion of a hormone that 'degrades' the 'perceived toxin' to a non-toxic metabolite. Which is to say that bitter compounds were perceived as toxic—most plant alkaloids are intensely bitter. So when the bitter receptors in the mouth and stomach release gastrin, we are assured of a rush of acid to nuke the supposed toxin. An atavism, but it serves to remind us that gastric acid is *defence*.

To hold it responsible as 'store-house and shop' is accusation enough—but does the stomach change its behaviour in obesity?

The vagus nerve is actually a double agent, dabbling with both ghrelin and leptin. When the vagus senses food in the stomach by a change in the tension of the muscle wall, it protests with an 'enough' signal. But that is quickly overtaken by ghrelin, and the silenced vagus sulks till leptin kicks in. Cutting the vagus nerve just below the diaphragm interrupts all nerve fibres to the stomach, causes anorexia, early satiation, and, consequently, weight loss.

Obese people are slower to attain satiation. They need a greater volume as well as more calories to say 'enough'.

In obesity the feeding-satiation balance in the brain is distorted. Also, the stomach becomes unreceptive to signals. For instance, many obese people continue to eat even when they already feel stuffed, almost as if they are unable to stop themselves.

Yes, the stomach undergoes a paradigm shift in obesity—but we don't know enough about this.

Too much gastric acid secretion?

Too much gastrin?

Too much somatostatin?

Increase in the gastric mucins that protect the wall from acid?

Up-regulation of genes that control gastric acid secretion?

Experimentally, two groups of obese mice—those that are genetically obese and those that have become obese on a high-fat diet—show changes in the expression of many genes associated with obesity, diabetes and insulin resistance. Most of these changes result in an increased gastric acid secretion, which is probably gastrin-mediated.

The dramatic weight loss after bariatric surgery might actually operate through this channel.

Sleeve gastrectomy removes over 80 per cent of gastrin producing cells. The consequences of this might run parallel with the chemical gastrectomy the world's dyspeptic population has undergone in the last twenty years on a diet of antacids, H_2 inhibitors, and proton pump inhibitors (PPIs). It is going to take a long while before we find out.

Helplessly, the stomach always bears the brunt. Its protests are gagged. Distended beyond endurance with food it doesn't want, churning unwillingly its whirlpool of acid, it transmits its discomforts to 'lesser muniments'.

'Lesser' only because they are not noticeable on the popular rebus of the body. They are really all powerful in the machinery of metabolism—the liver, the gall bladder, and the pancreas.

The Liver

The liver is a secretive organ. It is overworked and underpaid, but doesn't complain until the abuse gets really unbearable. *Then* it overturns its reputation and goes for the jugular, inventing new hells in every body system till we buckle. And when we do, the best we can wish for is a quick end.

The liver maintains glucose balance on a very tight leash. A meal rich in carbohydrates raises insulin levels. In response, the liver absorbs more glucose, and reduces its own production of glucose. This maintains a stable blood sugar level. In diabetes insulin is ineffective and the liver responds differently. Now, after a meal rich in carbohydrates, the liver absorbs less glucose, but continues to produce more. This, in turn, stimulates the pancreas to produce even more insulin—which fails to act.

Liver cells (hepatocytes) take up fats to synthesize triglycerides. They store triglycerides as oil droplets and package fats as very low density lipoproteins (VLDLs) to send them out into the circulation. They also use fats for energy, by burning them through the process called beta-oxidation.

Hepatocytes also manufacture fats from dietary carbohydrates and proteins—*so everything we eat in excess is converted into fat.*

Cholesterol, our popular nightmare, has a great deal to do with the liver. Very little of the body pool of cholesterol comes from dietary sources. Most of it is synthesized by the liver. Cholesterol in the diet isn't easily absorbed. It is a tedious process of hydrolysis, conversion to micelles, pick-up by a transporter molecule, and then re-esterification into chylomicrons—and at the end of it all, only 50 per cent of it is absorbed.

Much more cholesterol enters the intestine in bile secreted by the liver.

In the liver, cholesterol is the starter molecule for the synthesis of bile salts and acids—essentials for the digestion of fats.

Cholesterol, bile salts, phospholipids, all collude in the formation of gall stones.

Gall stones are hardened deposits of bile. They form within the gall bladder. They can set up inflammation (cholecystitis) and/or get impacted in the bile duct when the gall bladder contracts to squeeze out bile into the intestine. This causes a painful colic which may precipitate dangerous complications.

Gall stones and gall bladder inflammations are believed to be more common in obese women than in men.

'Fat Fertile Flatulent Female of Forty' was the convenient mnemonic used to profile the gall stone patient in old medical textbooks.

The link between obesity and gall stones is undeniable.

With increased absorption of dietary fats, greater synthesis of cholesterol in the liver makes the bile supersaturated with cholesterol, which then crystallizes out. The dietary pattern of most obese people stalls the recycling of bile for long periods, and encourages precipitation of cholesterol crystals.

Rapid weight loss is just as likely to cause gall stones—it is a common complication of 'crash diets', and of ill-planned bariatric surgery.

The liver plays a crucial role in protein metabolism as well. It 'de-aminates' amino acids, and converts their non-nitrogen components into glucose and fat. This is a very important function, so important, that any disturbance in it is diagnostic of liver disease. The 'liver enzymes' on the blood report, alanine transferase (SGPT) and asparate transferase (SGOT), are sensitive indicators of the state of health of the liver.

The liver is a major detoxifier. It removes dangerous ammonia by converting it into urea. Most of the toxins in food, and medicines, are rendered harmless by the indefatigable liver long before we get a chance to even notice them.

Many of the body's important proteins—albumin to begin with—are synthesized by the liver. Among these proteins are the essential clotting factors that keep us from bleeding to death from small cuts and bruises.

The magisterial liver is the éminence grise in all tantrums of the body, not just dyspeptic gall bladder disease.

More ominous though, is the silent change the liver undergoes in obesity. More than 80 per cent of people with obesity have a condition called Non-Alcoholic Fatty Disease of the Liver (NAFDL) which is just a grand manner of saying there is fat deposition.

So what, you said?

NAFDL carries with it some very dangerous corollaries.

Because of our propensity for Metabolic Syndrome, the Indian paunch is a sure sign of silent NAFDL. Its complications are much higher here than in the West.

The process starts with a deficiency of the 'good adipokine' adiponectin. This discourages fat utilization and encourages fat deposition in the liver. The process of fat deposition is accompanied by the inflammatory reaction characteristic of Metabolic Syndrome. In the liver, the principal inflammatory cells are Kupffer cells, also known as stellate macrophages.

This inflammatory state is the starting point for more lasting damage—the actual death of hepatocytes and their replacement with fibrous tissue. This condition is called Non-Alcoholic-Steato-Hepatitis, commonly referred to as NASH, and is really very bad news.

NASH is associated with a high degree of insulin resistance and high circulating insulin levels—both typical of Metabolic Syndrome.

The vexed question pops up again. Which came first? NASH or insulin resistance?

It isn't very clear why some people with NAFDL go on to develop NASH, while others do not. The answer seems to lie in two hypotheses.

The first is insulin resistance.

The second involves mitochondria. Beta-oxidation of fats is a mitochondrial activity, and when there is an overload, anti-oxidants like glutathione and Vitamin E are simply not enough to combat the build-up of Reactive Oxygen Species

(ROS). This leads to mitochondrial damage and eventual cell death.

Does NAFDL improve with weight loss?

It does.

What about NASH?

The outlook is guardedly optimistic. The caution is advised because the known danger of NASH is cirrhosis, with its looming horrors of liver failure and cancer.

In the damage that obesity can inflict on the liver, the chief conspirator is the disordered microbiome.

Changes in the microbiome have been invariably noted in obesity and Metabolic Syndrome. Again, as usual, the jury is still out on which came first. But it is worthwhile checking on the nature of mischief.

High caloric diets alter the microbiome. This 'obesogenic' microbiome alters the intestinal degradation of carbohydrates to produce short-chain fatty acids, like butyrates which step up enzymes that encourage the liver to synthesize more fat (lipogenesis) and more glucose from the dietary excess.

The altered microbiome encourages lipoprotein lipase which makes the liver and the adipose tissue take in more free fatty acids, and increase the secretion of VLDLs.

The revised bacterial population in the intestine makes it more permeable to toxins. The liver, alerted to this, responds with active inflammation.

The stage is set for NASH.

The pancreas also maintains omertà and colludes with the liver in the metabolic disasters of obesity. Local inflammation and the deposition of fat (pancreatic steatosis) cause cell destruction. The overall picture of insulin resistance and hyperinsulinemia in Metabolic Syndrome leads irrevocably to diabetes.

And so the body politic conspires against the stomach to mount a coup d'etat of Metabolic Syndrome in obesity.

'You shouldn't have started it off in the first place' these lesser muniments shrug.

The brain, in its ivory tower, gives not a damn, as long as it keeps getting its fix of sugar.

It all comes back to the stomach, and what shall we do about that?

First, we must concede the problem, as it relates to the Indian stomach hiding within the Indian paunch.

Second, we must examine the crucial question: *Why* is this happening to us *now?*

And that will get us, almost reflexively, to the third step—the finding of solutions.

Our Steed the Leg

A five-mile gallop on shank's mare every day is the quickest way to health.

As dawn breaks over the city, the parks are filled with earnest exercisers, there is a gym on every street, and yet, there is no change in the 'obesity profile' of the neighbourhood.

On my street, committed walkers plod the circuit. Observed over six months, they seemed to fall easily into four groups:

The fit, who got fitter.

The overweight, without a visibly large paunch, who looked thinner.

The mildly overweight with visible paunch who looked thinner but still kept the paunch.

The obese, who stayed unchanged.

They are all total strangers, and their medical history is unknown to me, but their joy is infectious as we exchange a cheery good morning. They radiate a sense of well being.

Later in the day, this sours mildly into a sense of virtue. By sundown they will be giving advice. Dawn will find them urging karela juice and wheatgrass on me.

All of them, including those visibly over 100 kg, are feeling good at the end of an hour's exercise.

Is that merely the endorphin high that exercise so reliably produces? Is it something that has altered the metabolic state?

What do muscles have to do with metabolism?

Muscle has 'metabolic flexibility'. This lovely phrase describes a hybrid that can switch fuels. After a feast, in a high-insulin state, muscle motors on glucose. While fasting, in a low low-insulin state, it switches to fats for energy.

Where does this fat come from? Obviously, in the fasting state, circulating dietary fats are low, so it has to come from the muscle's own stores.

Muscle stores fat, as triglyceride.

As usual, we have to rely on our evolutionary cousin, the rat, to get a glimpse of how this works.

Rat muscle's content of triglyceride rises when there is insulin resistance. How does that translate to the human situation?

Voluntary muscle is the thick contractile tissue we identify as muscle on the gym poster. We also have *in*voluntary muscle in the gut and other body tubes. The heart muscle, also involuntary, has unique electrical and contractile properties. But it is voluntary or skeletal muscle that, from sheer bulk, uses up 40 per cent of the day's energy. To begin with, muscle is the body's largest insulin-sensitive tissue, and this makes it, practically, a glucose sponge.

Insulin acts by activating a glucose transporter protein (GLUT-4) which usually naps inside the muscle cell. Woken up, GLUT-4 hurries to the cell membrane and grabs every passing molecule of glucose, drags it in, and lines it up on the production line for breakdown into ATP.

As elsewhere in the body, this process involves dozens of molecules for both transport and transformation. Without insulin, on both the adipocyte and muscle cell, only 5 per cent of GLUT-4 is available on the cell membrane for glucose to latch on to. Under insulin's beneficence, this shoots up to 50 per cent.

Think muscle, and you think contraction, the tensing up of a soft surface—flat or curved—into a compact slab or ball spring-loaded for action. The word 'contraction' does not necessarily mean a reduction in muscle dimension. It is more correct to think of it as muscle 'tension'.

When individual muscle fibres tense up, the muscle contracts. When a muscle relaxes, the fibres return to their resting state.

This special attribute of muscle is because its fibres contain filaments of two proteins, actin and myosin, interlocked in a sliding mechanism that allows development of tension with or without a change in length. The T-tubule system is a very special part of the muscle cell. This is a network of fine tubules that are inward projections of the cell membrane. The T-tubules are primarily responsible for initiating contractility in muscle protein on nerve stimulation. They are also responsible for translocation of glucose brought in by GLUT-4.

With repeated exercise, a physiological adaptation is achieved. This simply means—everything works better. As you train, it takes more, and longer, to feel fatigue.

Muscle is powered by oxygen. Oxygen consumption jumps up dramatically during exercise to provide ATP from glucose and fat.

The two types of exercise—aerobic (endurance) and resistance—impose different demands on muscle. The first is high frequency activity without an increase in load. The second is increasing load at a low frequency.

Insulin sensitivity increases during exercise and stays high for 48 hours thereafter. In obesity, this is impaired. This has been directly related to the amount of cholesterol in the cell membrane and T-tubules.

With the onset of obesity, there is cholesterol deposition in muscle. As the cholesterol in the cell membrane increases, the transport of GLUT-4 is impaired, and reduces glucose availability. The critical factor that determines insulin resistance seems to be the cholesterol in the cell membrane and T-tubules.

During exercise, muscle uses energy from its own stores, as well as from nutrients in the circulation. How much and where from, depend on the demands of exercise.

During mild or moderate aerobic exercise, muscles utilize glucose in the circulation. This comes from the last meal eaten, or from the liver which has synthesized glucose from fatty acids liberated by adipose tissue. This is under hormonal control; insulin and adrenergic nerves play against each other for metabolic balance.

As exercise intensity increases, fatty acids step back and muscles power entirely on glucose, till at peak, they draw on their own store of sugar (muscle glycogen).

As exercise continues, usually after an hour or so, muscles switch back to fatty acids from the circulation, and oxidize them for energy.

Muscle stores of fat (intramuscular triglyceride) are brought into play when exercise is prolonged further (over ninety minutes).

In exercise against resistance, the local sources of glucose and fats are utilized as usual, but controls on the supply of glucose and fat from the circulation are still hazy.

In both forms of exercise, 5–15 per cent of the energy is also drawn from protein. Muscle protein degradation supplies the amino acids for this.

After exercise, the body tries to recover by replenishing muscle stores of glycogen, so it switches again to burning fats for energy.

It takes 24–48 hours to recover all the muscle glycogen and fat used up during prolonged and heavy exercise. Dietary nutrients pull this off, under the guidance of insulin. A high-sugar-high-fat meal overcompensates, and establishes energy excess. That pleasant hour in the coffee shop after a great workout will do just that.

Exercise activates critical genes. They liberate chemicals that act on muscles and influence energy balance. Aerobic exercise, which increases mitochondrial activity, is cardio-protective. Exercise against resistance bulks up muscle mass.

Exercise has an overall insulin-like action on muscle. A cheery thought, because this suggests an insulin-independent path for glucose metabolism. Yes, there is some other magic that can get glucose into the cell. Peroxisome proliferator-activated receptor γ coactivator 1-alpha (PGC-1γ) stimulates GLUT-4 expression. It increases mitochondrial activity and so enhances both fat and glucose metabolism. Exercise increases muscle content of PGC-1γ.

Exercise also encourages fat metabolism. Fatty acid transporter proteins are activated by exercise, this results in greater oxidation of fats for energy, and a fall in circulating levels of fat.

Muscle also secretes chemicals, myokines, that have both local and distant effects, in much the same manner as adipokines do. For instance, insulin secretion from the pancreas can be inhibited by myokines from muscles which are insulin-resistant in obesity, but not by myokines from insulin-sensitive muscle.

The role of muscle in metabolic balance is turning out to be far more complex than we earlier believed. How does this change in obesity?

In obesity, muscle loses its metabolic flexibility because of insulin resistance. In the presence of high circulating levels of insulin, it can no longer utilize sugar for energy, although fat oxidation continues as before. When insulin resistance abates with weight loss, this flexibility is restored.

Once obesity has set in, the accumulation of fat in the muscle cell leads to increased oxidative stress and an accumulation of damaging Reactive Oxygen Species (ROS).

Moderate exercise can improve the metabolic status in obesity, but on its own, without addressing the disordered nutrition, it can do little to promote fat loss.

In the obese, intensive exercise comes with a clear and present danger of cardiac strain.

What happens when physical activity is reduced to the bare minimum of chair-to-bathroom-and-back through most of the waking day?

First, large blocks of muscle, in the back and lower extremities simply twiddle their thumbs, and do no work at all. And the muscles that are put to work face a lack of lipoprotein lipase, the enzyme which frees fat from triglycerides so that they can enter the cell for oxidation to produce energy. It isn't very clear *why* this important enzyme should slack off, but the consequences are predictable: reduced uptake of fats from the circulation, rising serum triglycerides, a fall in HDL, and—of course, obesity. During even short periods of exercise, lipoprotein lipase increases in skeletal muscle to free fatty acids for rapid oxidation. Muscle contraction up-regulates the release of this enzyme, and physical inactivity down-regulates it.

It is becoming apparent that inactivity is more than a default position. It has its own metabolic agenda that might do actual harm.

Changes in muscle metabolism during and after exercise mirror an ancient memory.

Our ancestors, who lacked our facility for three square meals a day, often had to trek miles to find lunch. Feasts were likely to be followed by lean periods when prey eluded them. Droughts and other hardships made fruit and berries scarce, and famine seemed always just round the corner. Accordingly, body stores of energy had to be optimized.

A thrifty genetic selection opted for a metabolic shift: during feasting, muscle powered itself on glucose. When lean times came around, fat became the fuel of choice. And, in the interim, muscle stores of glycogen were replenished.

This theory of thrifty genes was advanced by the geneticist James van Gundia Neel in 1962, as an explanation for the emergence of diabetes. He postulated that as cycles of feasting/fasting no longer prevail in our species, the thrifty metabolic shift precipitates diabetes.

In the past fifty years, Neel's theory has come full circle. After being dismissed at the end of the last century, it is now bright with promise as a likely explanation for obesity and Metabolic Syndrome.

The present idea is that these thrifty genes worked well at a high level of physical activity, and now that our species has turned sedentary, the expression of these thrifty genes is disrupted.

Instead of feasting/fasting, if we were to read exercise/rest, this theory seems to hold.

Glycogen is muscle fuel when intense exercise exceeds maximum oxygen uptake. When glycogen is depleted, muscle fatigue sets in, to make us feel stiff and sore.

What of 'weakness'—the feeling of exhaustion obese people commonly feel on increased physical activity?

There are several self-evident reasons—the excessive body weight strains anti-gravity muscles because of the increased load. We saw, earlier, that depots of adiposity secrete pro-inflammatory chemicals. This maintains a state of inflammation throughout the body, and especially in the muscles.

Muscle has satellite stem cells responsible for repair and secretion of myokines.

In obese mice, due to fat overload, these satellite cells become dysfunctional. Perhaps this is true in the human situation as well.

However, there may be another stronger, and more serious, reason. The chronic inflammation causes protein destruction within the muscle. This reduces the number of muscle fibres, and therefore, muscle bulk and strength.

Muscle misbehaves in obesity, contributes to 'weakness', faulty balance, and the joint problems that follow in consequence.

And the blame comes right back at...*the cormorant belly, who is the sink o' the body.*

Shadow Play—The Microbiome

We became aware, earlier in this book, of our body's second self, the *microbiome*. It is also the brain's most trustworthy espionage network. Not only does it transmit information about the state of the intestine, but it guarantees solutions as well. It is, in fact, the only protection the brain has.

'No way!'

Your outrage is justified.

The brain is our most delicate and precious body part. Unthinkable then, that the state of its health and function should depend upon a trillion germs lurking in our portable toilet.

Such, though, is the truth.

Disorders of the brain which terrify us—Alzheimer's, Parkinson's, mental illnesses that subvert the joys of life—all of these are linked to a sick microbiome.

Incredible isn't it, that illnesses so far removed and unconnected with our digestive tract should have links with the gut microbiome?

The evidence lies in the Microbiome-Gut-Brain-Axis.

And, considering the provenance, the evidence lies in our food.

First, consider the microbiome itself. How did we acquire these germs?

Within moments after birth, we welcome bacteria into all parts of our body. When a baby is weaned, the bacterial flora of the intestine changes and becomes more diverse. By early childhood, diet begins to decide the diversity and quality of the microbiome. In adulthood, our daily dietary decisions contribute in every way to the maintenance of a healthy microbiome.

We met the principals in the microbiome earlier, Bacteroidetes and Firmicutes.

We saw too that this is a loose, arbitrary division. Data suggests that the microbiome may be as personalized as a fingerprint. Nonetheless, there are some broad categories that apply.

Ultra-processed foods—which safely include all packaged foods, all bakery goods, and a good deal of gourmet delicatessen—give rise to 'dysbiosis'*—a deranged gut microbiome.

The ultra-processed foods are largely high-sugar and/or high-fat, low-fibre foods based on refined carbohydrates like maida.

Forget bacterial changes involved in the microbiome, what is the human experience of dysbiosis? What does it do to us?

Just about everything, apparently. It can precipitate Metabolic Syndrome, diabetes, heart disease, hormonal problems—not to mention a zillion discomforts relating to digestion itself.

Besides the ultra-processed food we gorge on, environmental toxins, those POPs so plentiful in food, and the unwise use of antibiotics, all these contribute to dysbiosis.

Dysbiosis alters intestinal permeability. This boasts a very dramatic label that I prefer to avoid because of the bizarre and misleading picture it conjures up. The intestinal lining with its tightly packed cells and their protective secretions creates an effective barrier when the microbiome is healthy. In dysbiosis, this barrier is no longer effective.

*Also sometimes called dysbacteriosis.

This happens because ultra-processed foods encourage overgrowth of the wrong sort of bacteria and the accumulation of lipopolysaccharides (endotoxins, secreted by bacteria) which stimulate the production of inflammatory chemicals, and cause local immune reactions that alter intestinal movements and permeability. This produces symptoms—painful cramps and diarrhoea or constipation—very similar to those attributed to food 'sensitivities' or intolerance.

Stress-induced bowel problems like Irritable Bowel Syndrome come about this same manner.

It is now evident that dysbiosis alters the Blood-Brain-Barrier by making it more permeable. This translates in the brain as glial inflammation, often a stepping-stone to neurodegenerative disease.

How does the gut microbiome link up with the brain?

Readers will probably answer that correctly with: 'In the usual way.' By now, we have followed the body's various modes of communication: through the blood, through nerves, through signalling molecules. These are the usual ways and the Microbiome-Gut-Brain Axis employs all of them.

Information from the intestine is relayed via the nerves in its wall to the vagus nerve and thence to the brain. Vagal receptors also sense leptin and ghrelin levels. The contents of the meal—fats, carbohydrates, proteins—are announced to the brain. Cells in the intestinal wall, neuroendocrine cells, secrete local hormones, of which more than sixty are known. Ghrelin, leptin and CCK garner the most headlines.

Not to be outdone, the brain responds through the Hypothalamic-Pituitary-Adrenal axis and the vagus nerve.

The intestinal cells produce neurotransmitters too: serotonin, melatonin, gamma-aminobutyric acid, histamines and acetylcholine. These alter intestinal rhythm and movements which we perceive with varying degrees of discomfort.

Can dysbiosis be corrected, and the normal microbiome be restored?

Thankfully, yes, and very easily so.

Vegetables and fruits provide the necessary fibre which cultivates the right kind of bacteria. That hoary 'anti-oxidant' mantra of polyphenols also operates more overtly by changing the intestinal bacteria. As the bacterial population diversifies, short-chain fatty acids produced by the microbes increase. These short-chain fatty acids are acetate, butyrate and propionate.

Acetate and butyrate are related to ketones, and are considered neuro-protective.

Propionate is absorbed by the liver and increases insulin sensitivity.

Butyrate, which provides energy to intestinal cells, also blocks inflammation.

Most bowel disorders and indeed most neurological disorders have a backstory of chronic inflammation caused by dysbiosis.

How does dysbiosis cause obesity?

Gut slime, politely termed mucus, may be a key player.

The right sort of bacteria degrade mucus to compounds that increase satiation, improve lipid metabolism and accumulate short-chain fatty acids.

The wrong bacteria do just the opposite. They alter bowel permeability by inducing inflammation and produce endotoxins. Endotoxemia is known to increase insulin and leptin resistance. More, local changes in the immune cell population releases factors that encourage deposition in fat depots.

The Indian traditional diet (caste/community/creed/geography/language are absolutely no bar) has the basics just right: plenty of fruit and vegetables, cereals fermented and unfermented, dairy.

We ought to be eubiotic and obesity free as a nation. What base treachery made us fat?

High Blood Pressure

The first meta-analysis of the association between obesity, hypertension and type 2 diabetes mellitus (T2DM) among adults in India was announced in January 2018. It examined published reports between January 1980 and January 2016. The conclusions were predictable. There is an indisputable link between hypertension and obesity. These are self-evident facts, but often it requires statistics to enforce health policy.

How will this very important and intelligent analysis, if at all, impact our nation?

Another study, this one about the prevalence of hypertension in North India surveyed more than 5,000 people and found 40.1 per cent with high blood pressure. Of these, only 30 per cent had been previously diagnosed as hypertensive. Startling, to say the least.

Undiagnosed hypertension is commoner than we think in over-weight people. It is also common in a much younger age group. No surprise then to encounter hypertension in a young man of twenty-five with a BMI of 30.

At twenty-five? When life's obstacles and disappointments should be very far away? When the strength to move mountains and to roam beyond the stars are your domain? High blood pressure? Now?

What does it mean, exactly, this diagnosis of *hypertension*?

Young people tend to misread this word. 'Chill' is the kindly advice their friends give them. The victim ascribes it to overwork. There is no such thing as overwork at twenty-five. So, what is happening in that 90-kg frame? Damaging changes in the heart and blood vessels which will lead to established cardiovascular disease, unless treated. Will prompt treatment at this stage reverse these changes?

We have known, for nearly fifty years, of the link between hypertension and obesity. And we have known about the dangers of obesity for even longer. What is left to discover? Every new study states the obvious afresh. Meanwhile, both obesity and hypertension continue to rise globally.

This note on high blood pressure is to highlight certain new, and alarming, observations. First, and most frightening, is the undiscovered—a large portion of the world's population has undiagnosed, and therefore, *untreated* hypertension. No matter how young you are, if you are overweight, please get a blood-pressure check.

Second, people with acceptable body weight and diagnosed with hypertension have a tendency to rapid weight gain. Not only does obesity lead in to hypertension, but population studies show that hypertension encourages obesity. That is a neat circle of evil.

Third, obesity fosters and hastens the truly crippling complications of hypertension: kidney and cardiovascular disasters. Obesity causes structural damage which soon becomes irreversible.

Fourth, women are at particular risk. Before menopause, oestrogen protects the cardiovascular system. In obesity, this protective effect is lost. It is even more ineffectual once Metabolic Syndrome is established, and it is practically non-existent in diabetes. Cardiovascular disease has been wrongly gendered as being male. There are more women with undiagnosed high blood pressure and heart disease. Obese women are more susceptible to these complications than are men of similar BMI. Also worth noting is that obesity in both parents is associated with childhood obesity.

Commercially preserved foods have two dangerous ingredients that not only raise blood pressure, but cause kidney damage:

- *fructose* from corn syrup used as a sweetener and emulsifier, and
- high amounts of salt.

Salt and fructose together are even more disastrous.

Even before high blood pressure is detectable, obesity causes arterial damage. Arteries begin to lose their elasticity. The muscle in their walls is damaged, and so is their inner lining (endothelium). These are related to the emergence of insulin resistance. At the molecular level, insulin resistance evokes a loss of muscle relaxation and the small blood vessels remain in a clench, increase peripheral resistance and cause high blood pressure. Leptin from adipose tissue is the strongest advocate of insulin resistance. So even if the blood pressure is not measurably high, obesity has already set the stage for cardiovascular damage.

Can this be reversed?

YES!

Fat loss invariably leads to a more stable blood pressure. Consequently, the dread complications of stroke, heart attacks and kidney failure can be held at bay.

A 'Civilization Syndrome'

In common parlance, the word *hormone* is an excuse, a whinge, a passing phase, as in 'It's just hormonal, I'll get over it.' It conveys a mercurial, treacherous state of being; temperamental, irrational, a fit of temporary insanity.

The truth is very different.

Hormones are constancy, precision, logic and reliability. When they're out of tune, among the many ills that seize us, the commonest is obesity.

The hormonal orchestra is philharmonic. Strings, woodwind, brass, percussion, keyboards are all represented, but their individual voices are swept up in sublime harmony. This is made possible by the conductor—and the concert master.

The conductor, as expected, is in the brain, a familiar part, the hypothalamus. Its Paraventricular Nucleus (PVN) to be precise. Its signals take the form of two hormones, Corticotrophin Releasing Hormone (CRH) and Arginine Vasopressin (AVP). These are conveyed to the rest of the orchestra by the concert master, the Hypothalamic Pituitary Adrenal (HPA) axis—which also tells the hypothalamus about what's going on in the pit.

Today we regard the HPA as the sensitive determinant of hormonal balance. When it is inattentive, there is discordance, chaos, and of course, obesity.

This is how the HPA axis works:

Hypothalamic CRH and AVP stimulate the pituitary into releasing Adrenocorticotropic Hormone (ACTH). As its name suggests, this in turn stimulates the cortex, the outer part of the adrenal glands,* into secreting corticosteroids, better called Glucocorticoids, because *they raise blood sugar*. This is the blueprint all medical textbooks have carried for a century.

Now, for the update.

Like *hormone*, the word *adrenaline* is also used casually, but here in quite the correct sense. It conveys stress.

Again, the colloquial use of 'stress' projects its meaning dramatically. One is never just stressed, but *stressed out*. That is a precipitous phrase. Beyond lies the abyss, but you're *pumping adrenaline*, and counting on that to get you across.

Adrenaline or epinephrine, or Epi as it is increasingly being called, is secreted by the medulla, or the inner part, of the adrenal glands.

Medical texts have fed us this 'fight-or-flight' function of adrenaline's since Harvard physiologist Walter Bradford Cannon described it in 1915. First-year medical students even today are still taught this atavism that describes the time when our remote ape ancestors faced off sabre-tooth tigers 11,000 years ago.

In 1974, Hans Selye† took a second look at stress and decided that 'fight-or-flight' could not fit our present circumstances. He proposed a three-phase response that reads like an epic novel.

Immediate adrenaline rush
General adaptation
Defeat and death

---

*These are also sometimes called the *suprarenal* glands, as they sit like jaunty little bonnets over the kidneys. The adjective renal comes from the Latin *renis* for kidney.

†János Hugo Bruno 'Hans' Selye (26 January 1907–16 October 1982).

Selye tapped unerringly into a scientific truth which we, in 2018, are still unable to swallow: *Stress causes disease.*

Twenty years later, it was accepted that when stress continues beyond a threshold, it results in a 'stress syndrome'—a collection of recognizably interconnected symptoms.

Does this mean our response to stress, any kind of stress, is non-specific and predictable?

Common sense tells us just the opposite. To be effective, the response to stress *must be* specific to the stressor.

How competent is our body's coping mechanism?

Even without stress, the body's needs are in a constant flux.

Think of it—metabolic balance, or homeostasis, cannot possibly be a stagnant state, and restore us always to the same point of stability. Life is constantly changing, and so are the body's responses. The adaptation of stability to change sounds paradoxical, but it is real enough to have a special name: *allostasis.*

This means a phasic re-setting of body controls in response to a challenge. It works well for the moment—but the long-term results aren't so smart. For instance, my muscles demand more energy when I walk uphill, and the glucose supply has to meet this demand. So, my heart has to pump harder. Luckily, my body's response is limited to the period of this particular demand. Beyond lies chaos. The polite term for this chaos is *allostatic load.*

Neither fight nor flight seems an appropriate response to the stresses of daily life. We merely endure them. So why do we need adrenaline?

Stress, to define it scientifically, is a state where an organism's homeostasis, or metabolic balance, is threatened. It is an alarm which brings the HPA axis into immediate attention, and changes the tempo of the symphony. The adaptations which are made before we can notice them involve the adrenals, the thyroid, the pancreas, the gut, the intestine, the sex glands—and of course, most importantly, the adipocyte.

The body's response to any kind of stress is an enhanced alertness, a sense of energy and purpose. Pain is ignored. Everything concentrates on the moment.

This immediate response is from the adrenal medulla which produces adrenaline. Glucose is spun out from every possible source. The liver manufactures more of it. Insulin is blocked, glucose doesn't enter peripheral tissues. Fat breaks down to supply more fuel to the liver factory.

All this is happening at the periphery. Adrenaline doesn't cross the B-B-B.

But the brain has its own adrenergic unit. It responds by increasing ACTH production from the pituitary which causes the adrenal cortex to secrete glucocorticoids.

This maintains the immediate response to stress, sustains high sugar levels and blocks off insulin until the threat has receded.

Only now does the HPA axis relent, ACTH backs off, and the adrenals stop producing more glucocorticoids. Insulin becomes free again to act and the stress response is over.

This stress response we exhibit goes beyond panic, fear, anger, concentration and rebuttal. We do not stick to a script, we ad lib our way into discomforts and crises. Panic can engender a heart attack. Apprehension can produce diarrhoea. Sadness and anguish can herald a migraine. The list is endless, and we have all been victims of it.

Today's urban lifestyle is a state of chronic stress, both psychosocially and biochemically. Under chronic stress, adaptation does not keep pace. We have junked the primitive fight-or-flight response, we are trapped in the system. What does our body do?

What happens when we neither fight nor flee the stress, but endure it?

That transforms stress into distress.

The first, and most universal, sign of life is the avoidance of distress.

The response to pain is our most primitive response, it is rooted in our unicellular past.

Distress is unnatural, unendurable, and life always fights it.

When it is impossible to fight, we resent it. Resentment breeds a deep visceral unhappiness. That is a very familiar emotional script.

Why should our physical response be any different?

This was first described by Per Björntorp as a *Civilization Syndrome*. This tag is all but forgotten, but it is better than *Lifestyle Disease* (which I usually mistake for an unreadable Sunday paper).

In 1993, Björntorp identified the following changes in Metabolic Syndrome and Visceral Obesity, and called these the 'defeat response':

'A twitchy HPA axis, leading to adrenergic overflow of cortisol, a damping of sex hormone response, increased visceral adipocyte response to corticosteroids and of course, insulin resistance.'

He identified the principal stressors as alcohol consumption, physical activity and smoking. He blamed this whole shebang on civilization.

Twenty-five years on, how does this read?

Cortisol increases deposition of fat in the abdomen, leading to Visceral Obesity. It also compels a desire for high-fat and high-sugar foods. In diseases of the pituitary and adrenals, when cortisol is dangerously high, the result is abdominal obesity and severe muscle wasting—cruelly caricatured in old medical text-books as the 'lemon on matchsticks'. Added to this is a life-threatening rise in blood pressure.

So, under the chronic stress of ultra-processed, high-energy foods, inescapable greed, physical inactivity, and, most importantly, poor sleep, aren't our cortisol levels always high?

Interestingly, the profile of glucocorticoids in chronic stress can be evaluated by examining scalp hair. Hair Cortisol Concentration is raised in various types of chronic stress. It is raised in obesity and Metabolic Syndrome, evidence enough to suggest a chronic elevation of cortisol.

The Hair Cortisol Concentration is highest in people with Visceral Obesity and Metabolic Syndrome.

Subcutaneous Obesity is not associated with high levels.

The HPA axis under pressure provides a circulating excess of epi, CRH and cortisol. CRH also releases a second hormone, aldosterone, which retains salt and raises blood pressure.

The kidney's special blood-pressure mechanism, the Renin-Angiotensin System is also under assault.

Glucocorticoids alter the immune response and increase the likelihood of auto-immune reactions.

The high glucocorticoid levels suppress the different hormonal axes—of the thyroid, of the growth hormone and of the gonadal hormone. This leads to loss of muscle and bone mass and, inescapably, the deposition of adiposity. Soon this culminates in visceral obesity, Metabolic Syndrome, and, eventually, diabetes. The fallout is cardiovascular, hepatic and renal.

In one word, ruin.

What about the steroid pills and injections we read about, on the sports page and elsewhere? Aren't they drugs that magic you way past wellness? Enhancers of every superhuman attribute? They're also very often prescription drugs. The truth about steroids is depressing.

Steroids are often prescribed unnecessarily, often swallowed unknowingly, and often marketed surreptitiously. Another old chestnut describes the consequences bluntly:

Steroids help the patient walk into the mortuary.

Visceral adipocytes have more glucocorticoid receptors and probably more expression of a second enzyme, 11β-Hydroxysteroid dehydrogenase Type I (11βHSD1) that retains cortisol in its active form.

Glucocorticoids disrupt sleep. Sleep deprivation increases ghrelin levels. We tend to raid the fridge when we cannot sleep.

Not surprisingly, crash diets stress the HPA axis out of its mind, and this results in weight gain as soon as you fall off the wagon.

Anhedonia, apathy, resignation and endurance all contribute to the distress of stress.

Stress seems to act at all levels of the HPA axis, from the brain to the adipocyte. It assures a milieu for visceral obesity, Metabolic Syndrome, then eventually, diabetes and cardiovascular disease.

Part 3

MELIORATIONS

The State of the Nation

One afternoon in 1978, I was confronted with cholera. I had never encountered the disease before, and the two children brought in with signs of this dread disease were very close to death. Luckily, they survived. Jubilant, I swaggered into the laboratory to crow over the enemy.

And there it was, a negligible punctuation mark, a squiggle of magenta on the pale high power field, *Vibrio choleræ Pacini,1844.*

I raced back to my textbook to see what it had been up to since 1844. The first thing I noticed when I opened the chapter was a world map with shipping routes. It was a cholera travelogue, and the main stops were detailed in the legend below, with mention of year and mortality in major European ports through all six pandemics between 1817 and 1923.

Nothing on that page mentioned India, except to say that the disease had originated in the Bay of Bengal. There was no mention that during this period, 23 million Indians had perished from the disease.

I slammed the tome shut, bludgeoned by its irrelevance.

What was the use of reading about elsewhere when I needed to know about the ground beneath my feet?

The newspaper this morning carried the *Lancet* study that links obesity and Metabolic Syndrome with a high incidence of cancer. A previous study on childhood obesity had also been noticed by the press. The reports voiced shock, more than concern and responsibility. It had taken the *Lancet* to make the newspaper notice that Indians are larger than ever before.

The truth is we do not, cannot, will not, see ourselves. Science is always happening *elsewhere.*

Here is some Indian data. It should alert those who refuse to trust what they see.

The India State-Level Disease Burden Initiative, published by the ICMR in November 2017, views the changing profile of disease, state-wise, from 1990 to 2016:

- Life expectancy has gone up from 58.3 to 70.3 for Indian men, and from 58.3 to 66.8 for Indian women
- Non-communicable diseases have increased in all states of India. Diabetes and heart disease lead the list.

In 1990, India had 26 million diabetics.

In 2016, India had 65 million diabetics.

In order of highest prevalence, India's diabetic states are:

Tamil Nadu:	>10.5/100
Kerala:	>10.5/100
Delhi:	>10.5/100
Karnataka:	9–10.4/100
Punjab:	9–10.4/100
Goa:	9–10.4/100

In 1990, 9 per cent of Indians over the age of twenty were overweight. In 2016, this figure jumped to 20.4 per cent.

Out of 100 overweight adults, 38 are diabetic.

The global average is 19.

To quote:

> The behavioural and metabolic risk factors associated with the rising burden of NCDs* have become quite prominent

*Non-communicable diseases.

in India. Dietary risks, which include diets low in fruit, vegetables, and whole grains, but high in salt and fat, were India's third leading risk factor, followed closely by high blood pressure and high blood sugar (high fasting plasma glucose). These risks drive health loss mainly from cardiovascular disease and diabetes, and also from cancer in the case of dietary risks.

Ours to Reason Why

A few months ago, I had a curious insight into India's scariest disease. I was at a medical conference, and the morning had been spent reviewing newer therapies for diabetes. The audience had drowsed through an hour of statistics, woken up briefly at the mention of a new molecule, and then relapsed into stupor until rescued by coffee.

The next session was on bariatric surgery for obesity, and the surgeon came in for some spirited heckling. When he returned to his seat, I overheard him say, 'If only they scheduled my paper after lunch—'

I never learnt why because he was abruptly cut off from view. At some silent signal, every man and woman in the hall sprang up in a single-minded lunge towards the exit. The aisle thundered with physicians and surgeons in mad stampede, elbows out, glazed eyes fixated on the door, pushing and squeezing their way out as if their lives depended on it.

Was it a fire? A bomb threat? Or all that coffee reminding them there were just two restrooms for two hundred?

Nothing so casual. This was a more existentialist crisis. It was lunch.

It took me more than half an hour to get to the food. Even then I had to fight my way past the phalanx queued up for seconds.

Everybody was eating everything: desi, Continental, Chinese, Italian, Middle Eastern, even something that looked coyly Japanese.

'So much better than the usual greasy samosa,' a diabetologist mumbled into his shawarma.

His wife shuddered delicately. Her plate held a small floury bun, dingy beneath a peeling eczema of oats and cracked wheat. The midsection oozed olive oil. She mopped up some more from a glistening puddle of shriveled fungi and fern, then swiftly speared a forkful of pasta before it could slither away.

'Extra virgin,' she confided, 'wouldn't touch it otherwise. I only eat Mediterranean.'

I wondered what kind of dessert they had served this polyphagic platoon.

'Ice cream, ras malai, Black Forest,' the chef hissed through clenched teeth. 'All gone in ten minutes.'

Suddenly, bariatric surgery seemed a great idea.

Back in the lecture hall, I found myself next to the Mediterranean.

'The figures have just come in,' she said to me breathlessly. 'Have you seen them? Shocking!'

She was referring to the International Diabetes Federation's newly updated 'Diabetes Atlas'. This eighth edition carries global data for 2017. The figures were indeed 8.8 per cent of the world's adults (18–79 yrs) have diabetes. That is 435 million people.

Most of them belong to countries that are either poor or developing, a slot India seems to permanently occupy.

By 2045, this figure will reach 629 million.

On the world map our subcontinent, dyed a deep blue, confessed to a 12 per cent incidence of diabetes. That means 72.9 million *diagnosed* Indian diabetics.

Sure, China was ahead of us, as in all else, with 114.4 million diabetics.

By 2045, India will have raced past China with 134.3 million diabetics.

I don't know about China, but judging from the past few hours, India is Usain Bolt-ing towards that goal.

The tea break, with its assortment of cakes and cookies, was an hour ahead. By the time the crowd dispersed after tea, each man and woman would have consumed two days' worth of calories.

Yes, dinner was yet to come.

And they had talked all day about how to tackle India's most frightening epidemic, diabetes.

How could they be so supremely unconscious of the irony? Their attitude revealed the schism we are unable to bridge. We are unable to translate what we know into what we do.

The thought kept me awake all night. The next morning on my usual walk, I deviated from the beaten path and walked to the beach instead. Dawn was still an hour away. The beach, now cleansed by a local philanthropist, was brightly lit with a row of ugly lamps. It was as crowded as a railway station, and nearly as busy. Only the sea lazed, the desultory tide dragging in garbage to uglify the wrack line. It might as well not have been there, that immense sheet of darkness crinkled with scatter from lamplight. Just another untraversable street. Pointless to glance that way.

Meanwhile, the sand tamped down by a thousand feet kept its resilience, challenging muscle, joint and sinew as people walked, jogged, sprinted, worked out, cavorted and cartwheeled, indefatigable like perpetual motion machines. With daylight, I could read the expressions on their faces. They were intent, committed, driven. There was no pleasure, not yet. That would come when the day's goal was met. It would power the rest of their day with a sense of achievement, and also a quiet pride at having met a responsibility.

The sun soon doused the sickly lamplight and the sea began to flex its muscles.

The first wave of ardently athletic young gave way to an older crowd—a much older bunch. The hour was wrong for young moms and dads, all madly rushing to get their kids to the school bus, then rushing all over again for their own harried commute to work. But these older walkers, forties and above, had the same concentration of endeavour as the teenagers who had brought in the day. In fact, their expressions were so alike, they could have passed for mildly battered clones. Their eyes were focussed on the next step, their conversations were sporadic. They could have been preparing for an exam. Nobody even glanced at the sea.

I knew who they were, all of them. They were all patients of the cardiologists I had been with yesterday—there was that certain separation of six degrees, but the connect was undeniable.

All these men and women were straining to responsibly follow good advice.

Among the older people, over half were considerably overweight, and most had the kind of paunch usually termed 'prosperous'. Sadly, this was true of many of the young people too.

For most of them six months on, little will have changed. That paunch will still strut ahead, no longer wobbly but ensconced in the dignity of a widened torso. Some of them, the younger ones particularly, will be considerably slimmer, but with that recalcitrant paunch still in evidence. They will soon regain their lost kilos, and then some.

And yet, nothing can be more desirable than this hour of intense physical exercise in fresh air.

Why is it going so wrong?

The answer lies, as always, in our national memory of food.

Contrary to popular belief, we didn't always eat at

home. People have always eaten 'outsidefood'—you had to, when you worked away from home. But 'outsidefood' was, generally, very like 'homefood'. And 'homefood', except on festive occasions, was plain fare: rice, daal, roti, fish or meat, vegetables. Milk, curds. Sweets were occasional treats. And those occasions were festivals or feasts. The food for each festival was unique.

(In India, religion is pure gustation, no matter how it is labelled. When it comes to guzzling festive food, we Indians are exemplar secularists.)

Gastronomic excess had a calendar all its own. These were notable meals, keenly anticipated, percipiently planned, and deeply relished. The menu seldom varied at these festivals. Successful dishes became tradition.

The description of the lavish meal in Ayurvedic texts isn't the daily fare of the impoverished physician or his students. Sushruta reminds us of this in his *Annapana vidhi vidhana.** An exhaustive list of confectionery and wines is followed by a directive of how such a menu should be served *to the king.*

The physician in attendance should see that the king first partakes of the sweet dishes, then of the acid and saline, and of the pungent and others at the end of the meal.

The king got his meal on platters of gold and silver, in bowls of crystal, glass and onyx, in 'fanciful trays spread out before him'. To his right, confectionary. To his left, soups, meat-essences, cordials, milk. And between these, innumerable bowls of relish.

The heavier meats arrived on gold platters, the more delicate dishes in silver bowls. Cool milk in copper pots, herbs and vegetables in stone vessels, wine in earthenware, and other dainties in small bowls of crystal and onyx.

The physician's meal is described somewhat differently: light, wholesome stuff with just adequate amounts of boiled

*The Rules of Gastronomy.

rice to be eaten, without haste, even when tormented by hunger.

So it appears that from the oldest records, royalty, however minor, had its special cuisine, and that simply did not percolate down to the hoi polloi.

The emperor Babar took great relish in describing meals in his diary, and two centuries later, Abul Fazl, that gastronome par excellence, revealed all the secrets of Akbar's kitchens. The emperor ate but once a day and never asked, 'What's for dinner?' much to his munshi's disappointment. The seraglio, on the other hand, kept its cooks on the run from dawn to dead of night.

Fast forward two centuries and you can revel in the decadent cuisine of Wajid Ali Shah. These accounts conjure up a past so luxurious that we can barely wait to claim it as our own. And claim it we can, in the repertoire of chefs, great and not, at restaurants, at take-aways, in DIY packets, and at home.

Every day now, we eat like kings.

The ingredients are not necessarily exotic, but where luxuries were once a garnish, they now permeate the dish. Almonds, walnuts, pistachios, apricots, once savoured in slivers that whispered of Samarqand and Kabul, are now ground in fistfuls into every gravy. Samarqand and Kabul, ad interim, are pulverized by the machinery of hate and the callousness of greed that crushes delight into a characterless paste. Where's the difference?

Dairy's coagula, once the purview of confectioners, now pop up in every dish on the menu. The glass of milk or lassi, the katori of dahi are déclassé. Instead, khoya and paneer, concentrates both, clog even our simplest dish.

All this is home-grown (home-groan?) stuff, I haven't gone global yet.

Almost all dishes on a restaurant menu will feature the stuff listed above—with loads of an import we like to call our own special contribution to world cuisine—the chilli.

Chilli formed no part of Indian cuisine before the seventeenth century when its cruel sear on the palate replaced the intelligent warmth of ginger and pepper. Chilli, a quick growing shrub that fruits generously, was gratefully chosen over the finicky and expensive pepper. The 'feel good' factor of chilli was undeniable, it provided a decent whack of Vitamin C.

In 1520, Hernán Cortés deprived Moctezuma of his daily cup of chilli-spiked chocolatl and handed us the chilli. We're now addicted to it. Fine, if you enjoy getting your tastebuds nuked. But there is an inescapable consequence. More chilli means more of everything—especially fats. Cooking with a lot of chilli needs a lot of fat if the oral mucosa is to stand the onslaught.

Capsaicin, the chemical which fires up chilli has a local anaesthetic effect, and you need a little more of sugar, salt, acid, bitter, umami to taste anything at all past the burn on your tongue.

Don't believe me? Test it out!

Every cuisine the world over is now chilli-loaded. This means it is fat-loaded as well. Cooks know that a lot of chilli requires a lot of fat—usually oil. The heat of chilli permeates the dish as oil dissolves capsaicin and distributes it evenly. The unstated reason needs to be stated here: without that extra protective film of oil, the dish will be intolerably hot. Instead of that interesting flush, the irritant will blister and excoriate the delicate mucosa.

How much oil/fat does an Indian household consume?

Per capita use of edible oil per year is 14.4 kg, as computed by the edible oil industry.

National production cannot meet this demand, so we import thousands of tonnes of it.

14.4 kg/year works out to 39.45gm/day—which is, very nearly, 10 teaspoons or half a katori or two ladles full.

That is 355 kcal, 14.7 per cent of the average day's requirement of 2,400 kcal.

Which is very modest on the global scale, and is also obedient to the ICMR diktat.

And yet, and yet, the actual fat intake in urban households falls between 40 and 30 per cent of the day's energy intake.

Pause here for indignant protests.

I hear you, I hear you.

A family of three usually buys 2 kg of oil a month, how then did the researchers come up with this incredible figure?

First, chances are, that the family doesn't actually *buy* 2 kg of oil every month. That is a backtracked calculation because what they buy is a keg of 5, 10 or 15 kg which lasts forever.

And 'forever' is a very elastic term.

Going by 2 kg/month, that is 20 gm of oil per day per adult, which isn't so bad at all, and works out to 10 per cent of the day's energy requirement, which is way below recommended levels, and probably perfect for an obese nation.

Then how do I trot out that outrageous figure of 40 per cent?

The oil we buy is what nutritionists call 'visible oil'. Generally, the amounts of 'invisible fat' we consume every day far exceeds this.

A quick list of invisible fats on the kitchen shelf:

- Oil seeds. Spices. Nuts.

Check the fridge next.

- Milk. Milk products: Curds, buttermilk, butter, cheese, ice-cream, cream.

That still excludes the group with the greatest invisibility—SNACKS.

Yes, we are soaked in oil—and, at what cost?

Obesity.

Metabolic Syndrome.

Dyslipidemia.

Diabetes.

Cardiovascular Disease.

Cardiovascular Disease is the leading cause of death in India, so it is really worth our while seeing how insidiously our fat intake fosters and sustains obesity.

Like I said, the Indian mind recognizes two major food groups: 'homefood' and 'outsidefood'.

To most people it is incredible that homefood, with its halo of pious virtues, should contribute to disease.

Many of us actually avoid outsidefood. And yet we're obese.

Two factors collude here: disinformation and cooking methods.

The first, I think, is more important.

Over the past years I've discovered how little we know about what we eat. Certain groups (doctors lead this list) are actually empowered to impose their ignorance on the consumer. At the household level, the cook knows a great deal about providing her family with delicious meals, but very little about planning and content.

The blame lies wholly on the commercialization of nutrition.

Selling an idea to the consumer has only one goal: to increase consumption.

So far, we have looked at all the body mechanisms that are disordered in obesity. Now apply them to advertising.

In this commercial, a plump young woman ponders the consequences of eating three bowls of halwa. She holds a standard-sized dessert cup of 200 ml.

Per cup, that is 50–75 gm of semolina, 75–100 gm of sugar, and anything between 30-50 gm of ghee. Three cups make that 2,235 kcal. Add a tad more from nuts and raisins and *it matches her energy requirement for the entire day!*

For a further nutritional break up, that is: 100 gm of fat and 200 gm of carbohydrate.

Now consider the interaction between the woman and the omniscient voiceover:

The woman's anxieties relate to

a) Deprivation of pleasure: 'Will I have to eat oats for breakfast?'
b) Appearance: 'Will I have to do yoga in tight pants?'
c) Loss of social relevance: 'Will I have to stop wearing jeans and t-shirts and start wearing shalwar kameez?'
d) Depression: 'Will I have to spend the rest of my life in misery?'

Only this last anxiety has any relevance to her indulgence, but it is quickly glossed over.

Nothing of the sort is ever going happen, Omniscience assures her. Just make your halwa from our sooji, and indulge yourself!

'Guilt-free!' chuckles the woman with a roguish twinkle that wins her a sorority of viewers.

This magical sooji is, what else, the African millet, quinoa.

Marshall McLuhan's famous aphorism is usually quoted as: *The medium is the message*. He soon altered that to: The medium is the *massage*.

The object being massaged is, of course, the viewer's brain.

To quote: 'All media work us over completely. They are so pervasive in their personal, political, economic, aesthetic, psychological, moral, ethical, and social consequences that they leave no part of us untouched, unaffected, unaltered.'

This particular commercial taps into every known mechanism of Indian obesity.

To begin with, I know very few people who would ever eat three dessert cups of halwa at one go. But the ad presumes that it is the usual thing to do. The scene is cozy. The woman is alone. There is the added pleasure of secrecy.

Yes! thinks the viewer.

There is no escaping the equation here.

Three cups of halwa isn't greed. It is *normal.*

In obesity, satiation comes slowly, hesitantly, demanding more sugar, and more fat.

The woman in the ad confesses to three cups of halwa with dread—however trivial her reasons.

The voiceover speaks straight to her hypothalamus.

It tells her it takes three cups of halwa to satiate her.

She *needs* three cups.

Want has become *need*, leaving her *guilt free.*

All that's relevant is that she should feel good about eating three cups of halwa.

Greed without anxiety is the goal here, and she has achieved it with the magical sooji.

The power of this advertisement cannot be exaggerated, nor can the Machiavellian intelligence of its irresponsibility, for the next myth it co-opts is the most dangerous of all.

You don't need this ad (or this book) to know that three cups of halwa will make you fat. It is common sense. So the ad dodges this self-evident fact.

The woman's anxieties show her perception of obesity as a cosmetic condition. The ad does not argue with this, perpetuating the myth in the viewer's mind.

The ad, which is for a 'magic ingredient', overlooks the other ingredients that make up the dish. This is far more effective than argument because the implication is that the magic ingredient renders other ingredients of halwa harmless too.

This ensures that the average cook viewing the ad will make her next batch of halwa without a thought about the dollops of ghee it takes. We can only hope she restricts herself to eating one cup of halwa.

At a time when most people get their information about food from the 'wellness' industry, an ad like this can be downright dangerous.

It is a very popular ad too for all the right reasons: the woman is very 'normal' looking. She is untrammelled by a supporting cast. This is 'me time'—a hard-won right for most Indian women.

It is equally popular with men who see this woman as a 'good sport', unlike her controlling sisters entrapped in perpetual wife-dom.

Why do I choose this ad over dozens of others?

It also highlights the 'happening' element when it says: *This is quinoa's moment, oats is so yesterday.*

As oats did to some other grain a few years ago.

The selling line is precious. It makes the state of impending obesity a peril exclusive to the privileged.

And it greenlights greed.

We saw how the hypothalamus establishes an addictive state in obesity. We then need more of of sweets and fats to register taste, and the taste receptor signals don't match up to 'enough'. Instead, they induce and sustain an orexic response: satiation is postponed, and the only signal the brain understands is 'more'.

(The most graphic exposition of this moment is in Munshi Premchand's autobiography where he describes being alone with a chunk of gur. If you find the hypothalamus hard to understand, read Premchand again.)

To exploit this state of addiction is cruelty itself. By dragging in the sentiment of 'guilt', the ad places obesity and greed as a very human indulgence. By inference it also says, 'On your head be it.'

Imagine using that stance towards some other life-threatening illness, like cancer. Oh yes, I know a Health Minister recently made a public statement that cancer is the result of human wickedness, but this book is addressed to intelligent readers.

The woman who has eaten three bowls of halwa is now a joke. She typifies the attitude towards obesity which has kept it from being recognized for the killer it is.

a) She is funny because she is fat.
b) She is adorable because she is weak-willed.
c) She is cute because—what the hell!

Like I said, imagine taking that stance about cancer or tuberculosis. We don't joke about those diseases. That would be horrendous, right?

Is it acceptable to discredit the suffering of the obese? Why not ask someone is who is 100 kg or more?

Even today, and even among doctors, obesity is seen more as a cosmetic problem brought on by an excusable greed.

No magical grain is going to protect a person from caloric excess.

Nothing will, except caloric restriction.

And while the hypothalamus in *established obesity* is wired for addiction, this is not true of the non-obese brain. It still has its satiation mechanism intact.

In all countries with a memory of want, 'I eat because I can' is an entitlement, and India certainly proves it.

Experiments on rats and mice have shown how the orexic-anorexic setting of the Hypothalamic-Pituitary-Adrenal Axis is altered on a high-fat diet.

Why should we be any different?

Any idea of excess is firmly edited out of public consciousness. Serving sizes are gargantuan. Come with me to a popular joint that is serving Mumbai's most happening snack, Vada Pao Fondue.

The girl who has just ordered one looks about twenty-five. She is soon joined by a friend and her mother. The two young people are mildly overweight. The mom is obese. The vada pao fondue arrives. It is the usual batata vada wedged in a fluffy bun with a wedge of butter and a dab of garlicky chutney. But then, here is the fondue—200 gm of cheese melting in an equal amount of white wine.

In ten minutes the fondue pot is wiped clean, and a second one arrives.

The girls are ready for a third, but the mother protests, and they settle for a good giggle around a matka mojito.

That was (presuming the cheese was cheddar and mozzarella, the usual combination here)—104 gm of pure fat in the fondue alone, shared between the three of them.

The hour is 5.30 p.m.

This was just a snack.

Which brings me to the biggest contributor to obesity: The Snack.

We are a snack-happy nation. Nobody is really curious about what's for dinner (not even Akbar), but everybody sits up and takes notice when you mention a snack.

And, we do have the world's world's most thrilling repertoire of snacks.

While watching this vada pao fondue being relished, a numbing beat has been thrashing out a tattoo in my brain for the past half hour: Tatatatata ta/tatatata Ta/ tadumtadumtadum.

Suddenly the words slide into place:

Theirs not to reason why
Theirs not to make reply
Theirs but to do and die

And memory has me in a different place and time.

Eight o'clock on a misty Calcutta winter morning. Sunday. I am eight, drumming out the 'Charge of the Light Brigade' on the dining table.

'Funny how all the people in the story have something to do with knitting,' murmurs my mother, who is knitting.

'Balaclava?' My father's voice is muffled by the wall of newspaper. He has recently been awarded such a cap against icy bicycle rides.

'And Cardigan. And Raglan.'

It makes no sense to me, so I continue drumming, with words, this time.

Theirs not to reason why
Theirs not to make reply
Theirs but to do and die.

'State of the nation.' My father puts down the paper and repeats. 'State of the nation, god help us. Ours not to reason why, ours not to make reply—' And throwing down the paper angrily on the table, he leaves the room.

After all these years the moment makes complete sense to me.

Strangely, today is the 2nd of December, exactly 136 years to the day Tennyson wrote 'The Charge of the Light Brigade'.

No other poem quite captures the mindlessness of obedience so perfectly.

I remember how the argument went on late into afternoon that day.

'It was an army. If you disobeyed orders you got shot.'

'They all got shot. If one soldier had pointed out the idiocy of it, nobody would have died.'

'They couldn't all have been wrong, there were 600 of them!'

'If 50 million people do a foolish thing, it is still a foolish thing.'

It was a quote, but I thought it neat then; I still do.

It is ours to reason why.

It is ours to make reply, no matter how the medium massages our brains.

What worries me is the way that fondue will sneak into the weekend repertoire of the home cook. With very many cogent reasons. Why pay Rs 500 for something that's likely to give you the runs when it can be made in your own spotless kitchen at one-tenth the cost? There is always a thrill in trying out a new dish.

And then there is the truly base reason, mine. The most illogical and seductive of all—for the sheer joy of owning a perky little fondue pot.

And there! Exeunt outsidefood, enter homefood.

We must face this—90 per cent of obese Indians have grown obese eating homefood.

The most powerful person in any household is the cook, because what she puts on the plate is so much more than food. It is the entire construct of etiquette and acceptable behaviour. It is trust and love and loyalty. It enslaves you as nothing else can, and the last thing you ever want is freedom. The food could be simply awful, but you never notice. It is beyond reproach. It is satisfying. It is *homefood.*

You'll agree this is a tough thing to confront.

But unless homefood is shorn of its meta-magical aura, we are going to stay obese.

What is going wrong in Indian households?

We are a largely vegetarian nation. Those of us who eat meat and fish don't always eat them every day, nor in significant amounts. So we are, for purposes of argument, a vegetarian nation.

But our daily consumption of vegetables barely meets half the requirement. That is a statistical fact.

To this I add one more truth.

We don't cook our vegetables, we murder them.

How often are the vegetables we eat recognizable in texture and colour?

How often do they look as pretty as they did before they hit the stove?

Do they arrive on the plate in shrivelled spoonfuls?

What about texture? Tender and succulent? Crisp? Squishy? Unrecognizable?

What do we taste? Vegetable or masala?

Can we get past the overpowering gravy at all?

That gravy is more often a confit—cooked and rendered in a large dose of oil.

Vegetables take next to no oil to cook to tender and luscious perfection, so why do we use so much?

Again, the reason is memory.

We cook as our mothers did, and they as their mothers did.

Or so we like to imagine. Inheritance. Continuity. Tradition.

But consider how time has changed things. Fifty years ago, there were fewer nuclear households. Families were not just bigger, they were infinitely expansile. The Indian custom of hospitality meant no casual visitor could leave without a meal, no matter how modest the fare. Our traditional recipes catered to that necessity.

We don't always (or perhaps never) downscale the recipe. Besides, only the rare festive dish has fixed measurements. Everything else depends on the cook's judgment.

Cooking is a breeze now with all our gadgets and innovations. Speed and ease demand a lighter hand. Cooking techniques must adapt to circumstance, not numbingly repeat methods which were efficient in a bygone age.

Just as we are a vegetarian nation, we are a cereal-happy lot.

The choice of cereal has historically dictated the choice of cooking methods too.

Wheat abhors moisture, rice loves steam.

Wheat needs fat to combat its gumminess.

This has led to cooking methods that are largely steam-based in the south, and open-fire slow cooking in north Indian cuisine, a method that calls for more fat.

Modern stoves and utensils guarantee a more efficient heat transfer and cut down cooking time. Recipes that traditionally called for large amounts of oil or ghee can today be cooked with a fraction of that amount. We need to embrace this change.

Western ideas of meal planning are very different from ours. The modern European meal is protein based. The amount of meat in a standard American portion can feed an Indian family of four.

The Indian meal is carbohydrate based. Rice, wheat and daal are our staples. Should our recent epidemic of Metabolic Syndrome, obesity and diabetes be blamed on carbohydrates?

Popular Western diktats have health-conscious Indians shuddering over 'carbs'.

How can what we've eaten for centuries suddenly turn around and bite us with disease?

Yes, the 'Indian phenotype' of central obesity and low BMI *is* linked with a carbohydrate-based diet, but we seem unable to ask *which* carbohydrate. The answer glares at us everywhere we turn, but we refuse to acknowledge it.

Consider Tamil Nadu. It is the diabetes capital of India. Over the last decade, most insights on this Indian epidemic have emerged from Chennai. The numbers there for obesity are staggering. You don't need to visit the city to check this out.

Switch to a Tamil channel on TV and watch any of the many cooking shows. The chefs, excellent with traditional dishes, really go to town on the novelties: dairy, oils, nuts and maida.

Even if these dishes do not translate directly into the family meal, the message subtly alters the home cook's perception of what is hot and what is not. These ingredients are not alien to South Indian cooking—but they are traditionally kept to a minimum. Increasing their use also shifts cooking methods from the traditional 'steam-and-sauté' to the crisper, flakier, sexier 'fry-or-bake.' It also buys credence for the home meal by making it closer to 'outsidefood'.

What is outside food in Chennai? Oh, the usual:

Samosasrollssandwichespizzaspastachaatcakescookies breadsbiscuits.

The fancy quotient will vary, but what is the common denominator?

Wheat.

Not the aromatic warm-hearted atta that makes the hearty roti, but the odourless, tasteless, chalky white maida that makes our daily bread.

Here is a population with suspect genes and centuries of eating rice as a staple, with steaming as the basic cooking method, suddenly opting for a lot of maida. This decision is concurrent with an alarming increase in obesity and diabetes.

It is not just Chennai; the rest of the nation is also consuming unimaginable amounts of maida.

I got a bird's eye view of this just after Diwali.

My friendly neighbourhood general store usually sells about 20 kg of maida a month. This jumps to 100 kg during the festive season.

'That's nothing! People here don't cook anymore,' the owner told me. 'They buy all their mithai and farsan. But at my other store, in Kandivli, I sold more than 600 kg of maida this Diwali, and with that you can calculate the amount of sugar and ghee.'

It was a very intelligent comment on obesity from a man who was neither a physician nor a cook.

When you consider maida, ghee and sugar are a given. Heated together, they achieve the irresistible Maillard reaction and the delicious caramelized crust that defines crispness. Sure, you can get that with atta too. But with atta it will be hard, not crisp; tough, not brittle; chewy, not tender. Chefs, take your choice.

Maida is a no-brainer when it comes to delicacies, but why do we need it every day?

Texture and appearance apart, what makes maida work is—convenience.

When you're rushed, lazy, overworked, fatigued, or just can't-be-bothered, can anything be more convenient than a sandwich? You can stuff it with whatever you want, pack it anyhow, eat it anywhere, and serve it to anyone with teeth.

Take two slices of bread and there's a meal before you can blink. Hate that soft white sliced loaf as much as you will, it is difficult to survive without it.

The other Indian staple is the biscuit. We eat more

biscuits than any other nation, and calling them cookies isn't fooling anyone. It is just your local bakery maal in a fancy wrap.

Me, I'm all for convenience. I don't agree with the widespread view that what is wrong with maida is that it lacks bran. We get enough fibre from other sources. Besides, certain dishes do need very fine flour, and we've been eating them for centuries—so why should, all of a sudden, maida be so wrong?

That is because maida isn't just very finely milled and sieved wheat.

Try sieving atta through a very fine mesh and what rains down will still not look like maida.

Maida is *white*. It is wheat bleached out of recognition by the addition of a long list of avoidable chemicals—among them, alloxan.

Alloxan, as any medical undergraduate can tell you, is toxic to the beta cells of the pancreas that produce insulin.

There is a coda to this, a qualifying clause, that researchers are very quick to add.

Alloxan destroys insulin-producing cells in mice, but the human pancreas seems curiously resistant to it.

Oh yeah?

I know they are quoting two studies that have been lamely floating around for decades.

Another argument is common—there is no evidence of beta cell destruction in Type 2 Diabetes Mellitus since there is no lack of insulin.

I find these arguments specious.

If we are in the grip of a killer disease, and we are eating huge amounts of a food contaminated with a chemical that has the toxic potential to encourage this disease, then we should not be eating that food at all.

Besides alloxan, maida contains benzoyl peroxide, bromates, chlorides and other objectionable ingredients.

It might make you queasy to learn that it is also enriched with an amino acid sourced from human hair.

Bleached flour is banned in all European Union countries.

China banned it in 2011.

Countries where it is still sold, like the US, also sell unbleached all-purpose and pastry flours, leaving the choice to the consumer.

Why are *we* still eating bleached flour?

For the last ten years I've been worried enough to do two things. I've talked to flour manufacturers about putting unbleached maida on the market. And, I have learned to bake a decent loaf without maida.

Most flour companies aren't listening. Some do, but point out that the market won't accept maida that isn't dead white.

'Whiteness is a mark of our purity,' one of them told me modestly. 'Purity is important to Indians.'

As for my bread, it is lighter and fluffier than store-bought, but you won't like it if you prefer your bread dead white.

How many people would want their flour dead white if they knew it was making them sick? With the diabetes epidemic worsening, with obesity in every second household, isn't it time we boycotted bleached flour?

Maida's fall from grace has spawned a niche industry in baked goods that is a complete swindle—breads with a smidgen of whole grain flour marketed as 'whole wheat', 'multigrain' breads with a sprinkling of oats and millet on the crust, wholly inedible bricks that call for a saw at the breakfast table, and brown bread coloured with burnt bran and molasses.

High-end bakeries know that customers who OD on gateaux will also buy a loaf that looks like poxy pumice because it is good for the soul.

None of this is nutritionally superior to store-bought white, simply because, despite the fancy disguise, it still is mostly maida.

The answer lies in making the use of unbleached flour mandatory for the baking industry. That might compel flour manufacturers to start marketing it too. And the awareness will give people the opportunity to choose.

Will it contain India's obesity?

It may, and in an indirect manner. It will force people to realize that what is on their plate makes the difference between sickness and health.

This is a very big step. It places responsibility back where it properly belongs—with each of us. It restores to us a power we have long abdicated—the power of conscious choice.

Solutions

An epidemic is silly season for new therapies, new investigations, new fads. Instead of getting an abdominal CAT scan to display visceral fat deposits, try taking a closer look at what is stacked on your plate. Low glycemic rice? A pool of olive oil? Flax, spelt, quinoa, teff, steel-cut oats? We weren't a fat nation before we heard of these wonders. Do we really need them now?

Will that glass of wheatgrass or karela juice, that nostrum of jamun seed and methi sold at the park really add to the virtues of a thirty-minute walk? Perhaps it will, if swallowed by the tonne, but it will never counter your menu for the rest of the day.

Think about it. The only way to evade obesity is to stop evading responsibility for what we eat. There is no magic molecule on the horizon, no stem-cell injection, no enchanted grain or seed growing on the sly on an undiscovered mountaintop that will deliver us from blindness, paralysis, coronaries, gangrene, and the many other morbidities of obesity, Metabolic Syndrome and diabetes.

The last free lunch was so yesterday. Nowadays, we always pay.

The first thing we need to do is to acknowledge that obesity is not a state of mind, or a cosmetic problem, or a sign of greed and poor self-control. Obesity is a disease. This means it will not budge unless treated. And, it cannot be treated by you, yourself. If you're obese, step two is: *see your doctor.*

That is much smarter than strolling into the nearest lab, having a slew of blood tests, and coming away consoled that all of them are 'within normal range'.

'I'm totally within limits,' a friend told me happily the other day.

You could tell from a hundred yards away that she wasn't.

As long as the lab reports read normal, nothing will convince her to seek help. By the time she sees a doctor not only will she be several kilos heavier, but her metabolic profile may have changed as well.

Since it is irresponsible to get to that point, why not act earlier?

If you are overweight, the time to act is now, before you get obese.

Rapid weight loss, and the attraction offered by crash diets, is downright dangerous. It has a 'pendulum' effect. Most obese people know this to their peril—lose some, put on twice as much in the next six months. What most of us do not know is the damage this causes. Rapid loss of weight damages the liver, makes NASH a frightening possibility. It is also associated with a high degree of gall bladder problems. As for the rest—*just don't do it.*

If you've read this book with interest you know by now that 'losing weight' is not always synonymous with 'losing fat'. If your BMI is over 25, your maximum abdominal circumference over 90 cm (male) or 85 cm (female), you are no longer merely overweight, and you need to see a doctor.

If you are veering close to the mark, with a BMI of over 23, or if you are of 'normal weight', but have a visible paunch, keep reading.

Migrations

Most people eat two meals, sometimes three, away from home. This is determined not only by working hours, but by their commute, which in any metropolis can be brutal even very early in the day.

What kind of breakfast equips you best for this ordeal?

Very few people who leave home early can bring themselves to eat anything. Usually, it is a cup of tea with a biscuit or khari.

And here is the source of the day's problems. A long 8–10 hour fast since dinner last night, followed by no breakfast, has the insulin-adrenergic balance already shaky. Hunger is simply not noticed as the pressure to perform builds up—get ready, get the family ready, pack lunch boxes, drop the kids to school, catch that bus, catch that train, queue for a rickshaw—breakfast on top of all this? Kidding me, right?

Luckily for us, we are crowded with convenience foods. But we think them inconvenient. Now is the time to change. Grab a banana as you rush out of the house, eat it on the bus or train, and you'll be less likely to reach for a samosa or vada pao at 10 a.m.

Ditch your cardboardy cereal and opt for a traditional homemade one instead. A porridge takes only two minutes to prepare, and with fruit and milk, it makes a great start to your day. Do you know how many traditional porridge mixes the subcontinent has? Hundreds! And each one is delicious.

There is nothing like an egg, nature's perfect food, to deliver your morning shot of protein. But our vegetarian nation shudders at the very mention—even though an egg is at least as vegetarian as milk. If every Indian child could eat an egg for breakfast, we would be totally free of malnutrition. We impose our prejudices and terrors on innocents and starve them of the means to grow.

Again, as I have said before, we are a nation unmoved by the suffering of children. Perhaps that too contributes to this epidemic.

Our prevalent anaesthesia against pain has numbed us to pleasure too.

A simple step to correct this is to observe and experience the world around your morning commute. It will restore your relish—for your next meal, and for life.

Naturally, after that long haul that has wrung you limp, you need a snack.

Snacks

Snack is probably the most exciting word in India, caste and creed are no barrier here. Its very mention evokes a sparkle in the most phlegmatic and can bring an angry outburst to a sudden pause.

The commonest snack we reach for is—a biscuit.

We are a nation driven by biscuits.

If you've made a biscuit yourself, you'll know how much fat goes into the dough.

If you don't—take my word for it, or check it out. Most biscuits are made from maida. The 10 per cent 'healthy' ones, which contain whole grain/bran, also contain just as much fat.

Any country with an epidemic of obesity needs to ban biscuits. If you know the size of the market and the cut-throat competition, you know this means bloodshed, so it will not happen. Besides, I regard any ban as an insult to human intelligence.

What then?

As always, we can rely on free will.

All bakery products are a very bad idea if you are overweight. They contain the two ingredients guaranteed to encourage obesity—maida and fat. The fat in bakery products is usually shortening, margarine, which has a high level of trans fats.

The best method of choosing a snack is to get smart on what it is made up of. Not all of us are cooks, but why not find out what we're eating to make a better informed choice?

If you're clueless about food—great! This means you can commence the adventure of discovery with an open mind. There is no pursuit quite as pleasurable as this one, believe me!

Snacks are India's biggest paradox. They are considered 'light'—they are things that are eaten *between* meals. Most of these snacks are high caloric, often with a greater energy value than a home-cooked meal. Some, especially the traditional deep-fried treats like samosa, kachori, vada, are acknowledged as 'heavy', but are still earmarked for that space between meals. Yet, even a samosa (flour to fat 5:1 ratio, and then deep-fried) is an innocent compared to a bakery product.

The 'lightness' of a snack is evaluated by its crispness.

Surat's famous khari, which is mille-feuille par excellence, is the 'lightest' snack people know. It is difficult to refute this. A well-made khari is a thing of air, a bakery sprite, exquisitely light, crisp, flaky. Its flour to fat ratio varies between 2:1 and 3:1. The fat is the very best shortening—saturated and loaded with trans fats.

In an interesting study on snacks in Delhi, researchers made several cogent observations that deserve wider attention. The population surveyed belonged to low-income groups. The snacks examined were the staple North Indian namkeen, locally made, and though some were branded, others were sold in unlabelled plastic packets or glass jars. This is the quintessential scenario in every city.

The researchers sampled a wide variety of snacks: fat content ranged from 28.8 gm to 29.6 gm fat per 100 gm serving for 'packed' snacks and a much higher for 'open' snacks like freshly fried kachori. The sampled cooking oils were high in saturated fats and trans fats.

Vendors and cooks had a poor understanding of the health effects of fats, and expressed desire to change to more healthy cooking mediums, if quality could be maintained.

That last phrase is crucial—the customer is king.

The very fact that small businesses may be open to change, if supported, tells us how important health information is.

Small eateries have supplanted the domestic kitchen for a large part of the day, and these entrepreneurs make up a huge workforce that can be educated to provide cheap and nutritious food—and, anywhere in India, turn out something delicious.

Now consider the effects of eating a high-fat snack.

Not only is the fat in excess, but the satiety it provides guarantees that the next meal will be small, and severely limited in essential nutrients.

What if we were to consider a snack as a main meal?

Some snacks work well this way—and the key factor is protein.

A chaat with all its spicy tease and crisp seductions has a hearty soul of chhole—top-grade vegetable protein. Add a potato pattie and a racy salsa, and that is an entire meal.

Idli, with a good sambar, works the same way.

Choices abound, and the easy way to pick the right snack is to have some idea of what it contains and how it is prepared.

What about the crisp snacks India glories in?

All the whorly curly flaky fragments that crunch before they melt on the tongue?

Give them a miss—unless you have the time, and the expertise, to make them at home.

I am constantly stymied by this lack of curiosity towards what is on the plate. I see it as part of the anhedonia of obesity. In fact, more than half the obese people I know are plainly uninterested in food. Reviving this interest could be all important in addressing obesity.

Enjoyment begins with anticipation and curiosity, and why not start by finding out what you are about to eat? A touch on the phone screen or keyboard will tell you everything you need to know.

A lot of this lack of curiosity is based on a fear of over-eating. You would rather have a bland and awful meal so that you can be certain you don't eat too much. When pushed to it, you would rather skip a meal.

Eat!

Nothing, really, encourages obesity so much as skipping a meal.

Any attempt at energy deprivation brings about an adrenergic rush. Insulin, already quavering, is shouted down by the imperious demand of the brain for a constant inflow of glucose. And that simply results in an increase in circulating sugars and fats, overcompensation and increase of adiposity.

Hunger is your worst enemy if you are overweight, so EAT!

Eat at least three complete meals a day.

A complete meal is one where all the food groups are represented.

The one element in which Indian home meals fall dismally short is—protein. A packed lunch invariably skimps on it. Which is why 'roti and sabzi' is woefully inadequate for your daughter's lunchbox—and yours.

A good meal is a great deterrent to a large snack.

As for 'fasting'—whatever its spiritual merits—it is dangerous if you are overweight. It will lead to weight swings that will cause significant organ damage. *Just don't do it.*

Eggs!

Eggs are probably the most suspect food in India.

An egg is just as 'vegetarian' as milk.

Milk is the secretion of the modified sweat gland of a mammal.

An egg is the secretion of the ovary of a bird, its ovum, generally sold unfertilized. Commercially bought eggs are always unfertilized. Fertilized eggs are usually sold as 'desi'.

Eggs are premium food.

Elegant in design, intelligently packaged, quickly cooked in a million different ways, delicious, and simply bursting with nutrition—what's not to like?

And yet, 60 per cent of Indians will gag at the very thought of an egg.

Worse, they will keep their kids from eating the one food that can protect them from malnutrition and disease.

So, what's objectionable in an egg?

Let us avoid the commonest hurdle—eggs aren't 'allowed in my family'. That I cannot counter with rational argument.

Smell and texture?

It takes practically no time, but quite a bit of intelligence to cook an egg. Apply yours and you'll have an egg that's appetizing and delicious.

Still can't stand it? Forget it!

And yes, some people are allergic to eggs, the whites especially—and should avoid them.

There is also the rubbish passed off as traditional wisdom: Eggs are *heaty*.

Indian households still trade on concepts of 'hot and cold foods' without any understanding of these archaic terms.

Mediaeval medicine happens to be my hobbyhorse, so I'll argue you off your feet on that one some other time.

Right now, let science assure you that eating an egg will not stoke your hidden fires. Your heart won't pump harder, your temper won't rise, your body temperature will stay constant, your libido unchanged.

The one modern apprehension that criminalizes eggs is, in one word: CHOLESTEROL

Aren't eggs *risky*?

Most people seem to see a direct connection between an egg at breakfast and a mandatory coronary bypass within the year.

This is especially true among folk who enjoy eggs.

Crack that perfect porcelain exterior and look closer at what's inside.

Egg white is—no exaggeration here—liquid gold. Egg protein, albumin, is the gold standard against which all protein foods are judged.

That's 3.1 gm of first-class protein per egg. In a protein-starved nation, a life-saver.

So far, there have been no scientific objections to egg white.

The vexed bit is the yolk.

Egg yolk is interesting. Besides a big punch of carotenoids which make it look like liquid sunshine, it packs exciting stuff we're just beginning to understand. But as this book is about fat and its relationship with health, let us focus on the fat in egg yolk.

One egg yolk contains 4.8 to 5 gm of fat, of which only 1.5 gm is saturated—that's 30 per cent.

One teaspoon of butter has nearly the same amount of fat, but more than 75 per cent of it is saturated.

One egg yolk has 200 mg cholesterol.

A teaspoon of butter has 10.8 mg cholesterol.

These are the figures to make your heart quickstep, especially when the day's 'safe limit' for dietary cholesterol has been fixed as 300 mg. Even one egg begins to look dangerous, leave alone two.

People have panicked over egg yolk since the historic Framingham Study* (now in its seventieth year) showed a link between serum cholesterol and cardiovascular disease.

The study said nothing about egg yolks, but since yolks contain cholesterol, it was taken as a given that they raise serum cholesterol.

Since then, eggs have been married to heart attacks.

Like a long, miserable marriage, the yolk-heart attack story is embittered by rumour and misunderstanding.

Do egg yolks really raise blood cholesterol levels?

If they do, then yes, they're justly accused.

Let us examine the evidence as of 2018.

Only 25 per cent of serum cholesterol is derived from dietary cholesterol. The body manufactures the rest from caloric excess.

So an excess of sugar and fats in the diet contribute much more than swallowed cholesterol.

A 70-kg man's body manufactures 850 mg of cholesterol a day. This is controlled by a complicated bio-feedback mechanism which is tuned by cellular cholesterol.

To simplify, there is a predictive equation about how much serum cholesterol might change with an increase of dietary cholesterol.

It is estimated that with every 100 mg increase in dietary cholesterol, the serum cholesterol may rise by 2.1–2 mg/dl.

If we examine further, that figure begins to look different: dietary cholesterol raises both LDL and HDL cholesterol.

---

*Hajar, Rachel. 'Framingham Contribution to Cardiovascular Disease.' *Heart Views: The Official Journal of the Gulf Heart Association* 17.2 (2016): pp.78–81.

The risk of cardiovascular disease is predicted on the LDL : HDL ratio, and this seems unchanged.

More, everybody doesn't respond in the same manner to an increase in dietary cholesterol.

In 'hyper-responders', egg intake does increase serum LDL, but it changes LDL particles to the 'large' subclass which are considered 'heart safe'—not atherogenic. Oxidized LDL, considered dangerous, does not increase.

People of normal weight, or overweight people losing weight, do not show an increase in LDL.

Concomitantly, they may show a rise in HDL, again in large-particle HDL that's considered cardio-protective.

The LDL : HDL ratio is maintained.

Surprisingly, eggs increase all other 'good' HDL functions as well. This may also be from the magic molecules in yolk—phospholipids. These compounds have jawbreaker names: phosphatidylcholine and sphingomyelin. These regulate the dietary absorption of cholesterol and also control the gut's microbiome.

So what's the verdict?

If you don't have Metabolic Syndrome, an egg a day—or even two—will not increase your cardiovascular risk.

I'll simplify that to an easy practical measure.

Think of egg yolk as a teaspoon of fat—2/3 oil and 1/3 butter.

And the cholesterol?

Think about the HUGE amounts of cholesterol your body lands up making from samosa, daal makhni or birthday cake! Compared to that the fat in yolk is a mere tittle.

The benefits in an egg yolk far outweigh its putative hazards.

Egg yolk is, put bluntly, BRAIN STUFF.

DON'T deprive your child of an egg a day, even if you won't eat one yourself!

The Fat Check

People today rely heavily on 'blood tests'. These have great meta-magical value. Annual tests seem to confer great solace even without the faintest idea of what they mean. Like the meaningless rituals of religion, these tests have acquired a moral status. 'No red lines' is all the reprieve necessary to abet a headlong canter into disease. Illness invariably strikes despite these printouts of 'wellness'.

This attitude must be questioned.

Yes, tests are absolutely essential for evidentiary proof of the metabolic state. But do not forget the first and most obvious evidence of metabolic change in the body is fat gain. From there to the establishment of metabolic disease may take years, but all this while those accumulating adipocytes are stealthily wrecking the body.

If you are overweight, two tests are absolutely essential: Lipid profile, and blood sugar.

Look at the most vexed part of the blood report—Serum Lipids that predict cardiovascular risk.

'Total Cholesterol' doesn't mean much.

Cholesterol circulates in blood, and around cells, packaged as five important lipoproteins:

- Chlyomicrons
- Very Low Density Lipoproteins, VLDL
- Intermediate Density Lipoprotein,
- High Density Lipoprotein, HDL

The liver makes VLDL from dietary fat *and also from ANY absorbed caloric excess.*

After VLDL enters the blood, lipoprotein lipase converts it into LDL, the 'bad' cholesterol.

LDL enters the walls of capillaries, gets oxidized, encourages inflammation and prepares the scene for the formation of fatty streaks which are fat-laden macrophages called 'foam cells'. Fatty streaks go on to become atheroma—lipid plaques—that obstruct blood flow and encourage the formation of thrombi—blood clots.

LDL should remain below 100mg/dl.

HDL, the 'good' cholesterol represents a 'mop up' of harmful cholesterol delivered safely to the liver where it can be processed into bile.

However, the benefits of high HDL have recently been seriously questioned. The HDL/LDL ratio, so integral a part of lipid profiling, cannot be accepted as a safeguard any more.

Biomarkers, C-Reactive Protein and Apolipoprotein B, should be evaluated as part of the 'fat check'.

What About Alcohol?

Alcohol stands midway between sugar and fat in energy value: 1 gm of alcohol yields 7.1 calories.

A glass of red wine will provide 80 calories, as much as a banana, and a little more than the same volume of milk. That's also the equivalent of four teaspoons of sugar.

So does alcohol contribute to obesity?

Yes, in teenagers and young adults, drinking alcohol leads to obesity.

No, in adults, unless it is heavy or binge drinking.

Yes, in older people.

There seems to be a clear age variation in the way the body metabolizes alcohol.

Women are more prone to gain weight with moderate drinking.

Both men and women who increase their intake of alcohol over a period of time incline to obesity.

Beer has been consistently linked with weight gain.

A daily glass of wine, rich in polyphenols from the grape, has been declared a health benefit.

That said, look at how alcohol can impact metabolism. To cut a long story short, alcohol substitutes ethanol for fatty acids in the liver, so the oxidation of fats for energy is blocked, and fat begins to be deposited in the liver. This is dangerous, as it leads on to liver damage.

In obesity, the stage is already set for liver damage, and drinking alcohol is simply asking for trouble.

If you have Metabolic Syndrome, it is smart to avoid alcohol.

In India, social drinking is on the rise, especially among the very young—who are also showing an alarming rise in obesity.

I rest my case.

Diets!!!!!

That needed more than five exclamation marks. But I'm nothing if not moderate ...

The list of popular diets that have worked wonders and then fizzled out could fill libraries.

There is no one-size-fits-all 'diet'.

Walk!

Nothing can replace physical exercise.

Walking, swimming, dancing, or a sport.

Choose your activity and get cracking.

At work, get out of that chair every half an hour and move about, no matter how compelling your job. It will rid you of aches and pains and keep the titanium out of your joints.

What About Packaged Foods?

They look attractive on the supermarket shelf, and if you are overweight, leave them there.

This epidemic, like any other, can only be countered by making it a personal issue.

This isn't about lavishing compassion on a disadvantaged population a thousand miles away. This is happening in your household and mine, and, no matter what biochemical clues new research throws up, the disorder is based on unwise eating.

In obesity where too much is always too little, winning our first battle may lie in recovering our delight in the small pleasures of a simple meal.

The Pale Horseman

> And I looked, and behold a pale horse: and his name that sat on him was Death, and Hell followed with him.
>
> —Revelation 6:8 (King James Version)

I drive through the jungle every day at noon. It is a small strip of road connecting two thoroughfares. On one side are corporate buildings with extra-terrestrial names like *Galaxy Supreme* and *Evershine Cosmic*. On the other is *terra infirma*, a midden of garbage. Demolished huts still stand upright like decayed teeth, the submerged bones of abandoned vehicles are covered with bright fresh washing and, further up, new dwellings of tarp and tin struggle for survival.

The extra-terrestrials don't show themselves at all, but at this hour, when cars are bumper to bumper, the inhabitants of the midden gravely conduct the traffic: white bearded men with tired eyes, or sprightly youngsters ready with humorous repartee. Nonetheless, we keep the windows rolled up for fear of man-eaters.

In the season of nagging rain, when festering heaps of garbage in tamped down plastic has viruses shouting out gaily, there is more than one sort of man-eater about.

One afternoon I surprised a little girl in a blue skirt dancing alone in the rain. The jungle had her at its mercy—dengue, chikungunya, encephalitis, diarrhoeas, who knows what next, man-eaters, child-eaters all. The pale horseman was everywhere.

When I was her age, man-eaters were a real presence in my life. Mostly tigers. I met a few at the zoo, but more in the tales of that intrepid hunter Jim Corbett. The Himalayas, with their misty huddle of villages, seemed created just for this guy to turn up with his gun, build a machan, and dangle a goat as bait.

To my eight-year-old eyes, the unstated story was far more vivid. A craven bunch of villagers who needed this noble gora to save them from a tiger they had lived with all their lives. The happy ending had a picture of Corbett, jackbooted foot planted triumphantly on a stripy carcass, and a servile contingent cowering at one remove.

Since none of those books contained pictures, I must have imagined it all.

All Corbett's books had children stuffing themselves with halwa-poori. Now what exactly was that?

'There's halwa and then there's puri,' my mother stated, totally disdaining the hyphen.

That hyphen was everything. Without it, halwa, any halwa, no matter how delectable, was just a sweet, and puri a trifling dirigible. But with that hyphen, their conjunction became the stuff you battened on when man-eaters were on the prowl.

My mother's attempts at Corbett cuisine made even our cat look smug. What good would it do against a tiger?

I don't remember anything of Corbett's tigers, but I thought of his halwa-poori every day as I navigated the jungle.

And then, a week ago, an emergency took me down that road at 6 a.m.

The jungle is a very different place at dawn. Traffic ambles, people potter about, dogs settle down to investigate an itch in the middle of the road. One notices trees. And on cables overhead, crows consider the day.

At the corner is New Hindustan Chinesh, a sign that draws a smile most afternoons and leaves me wondering what's cooking behind its shuttered door. It was open this morning, and judging from the buzz, business was booming.

Chinese food at 6 in the morning?

I couldn't look past the wall of male backs to see what they were gobbling up with such gusto, but the misty air lacked the queasy accord instantly recognizable as Indian Chinese: charred garlic, burnt cabbage, vinegar and soy.

I had forgotten about New Hindustan Chinesh on my return journey, and so I was past it already when I breathed in a very different aroma.

Wheat. Syrup. Ghee.

Chinese?

I parked on the nearest dunghill and picked my way back disbelievingly.

Yes, my nose hadn't misled me. New Hindustan Chinesh was making a paratha—one enormous paratha, on a tawa three feet wide. And on the adjoining counter a cooling kadhai held a glowering red mound of halwa.

There was only one customer left, polishing his plastic plate by now, so the two cheery young chefs took time off to chat with me.

Salman and Usman are from Faizabad, and the giant paratha they sell is called, variously, Normal Paratha, Halwa Paratha, Halwa Puri—depending on the customer's level of ignorance.

'Wait—did you say halwa-puri?' I demand.

Salman shrugs. 'Sure, some folk call it that. Those who don't know much.'

Corbett slid naturally into that category.

After all these years, and far away from misty Kumaon—halwa-puri!

Salman tells me their day starts at 3 a.m. when he kneads the dough. There is very little of it left now. He gestures over his shoulder at a large tub where a puffy coil of dough glistens like a python. Usman, the sous chef, is in charge of the sooji halwa. He pats it down to a slab, a red-hot brick. Its redness is primal, dazzling.

Salman shows off his skills as he picks up the dough and twirls it with an expertise guaranteed to turn any pizzaiolo green with envy.

Usman, meanwhile, grabs a cup and dips it in a tin of 'ghee'. He pours this with a flourish and a generous puddle warms on the tawa, sizzling merrily as the paratha flops down in a perfect 1/4 inch thick circle.

'How long did it take you to learn to do that?'

'About two months.'

After another four measures of ghee, the paratha assumes its flaky gold perfection.

Usman tears off a quarter, scoops up some halwa and weighs it out—quarter kilo—to the gramme.

There are new customers. Two young women, eyeing the tawa uncertainly, and mentally measuring the cost.

'Half kilo,' one ventures.

'No, a little more this morning, seeing it is so misty,' Usman retorts. 'This will put some josh into the little ones before you pack them off to school.'

'Okay,' they decide after a whispered aside, 'we'll take it.'

Clutching my hot package, I bid goodbye to the boys. I think of the children in Corbett's books safely stuffing themselves with halwa-puri, and of the little girl in the blue skirt dancing, oblivious of danger, alone in the rain.

I'm loath to think science. It goes so against the simple joy of the moment. The boys tired and sleepy, but happy at the day's work well done. The young mothers excited at the thought of smuggling home an unexpected treat for their young—perhaps my little girl with the blue skirt is one of them.

Shorn of its bona fides, the transaction takes on a very different hue.

The boys have sold a product made of ingredients purchased in good faith. One kilo of maida and 500 gm of vanaspati 'ghee' to the paratha.

The maida is bleached with the worst batch of chemicals one can imagine, but the boys rely on it's 'quality'—*white and pure.*

The ghee is standard-issue vanaspati that may contain as much as 30 per cent trans fats.

The halwa's redness is beyond cochineal and annato, carmine, and amaranth. Even the synthetic allure of ponceau red, erythrocine, and citrus red pales before it.

The 'kesar' is very likely the crumble of vermillion sold in most small rural stores, indistinguishable from sindoor.

My memory is jogged into recollection of Fredrick Accum '... red sugar drops are usually coloured with the inferior kind of vermillion. This pigment is generally adulterated with red lead.'

I worry about mercury and lead.

It could be worse.

Yellow would have meant metanil yellow, toxic to the liver and the brain. Green may have been malachite green, a known carcinogen.

Ignorant of these horrors, the mothers are happy in the thought that something deliciously flaky, hot and sweet in the morning might keep their little ones from gorging on vada pao at the school gates two hours later. The children, I'm sure, will do both.

Vada pao's political career is temporarily on hold, but it still remains the most 'filling' snack on the street. Mothers see it as outsidefood—unless *they've* done the buying, as with this morning's paratha.

Mother-bought, consumed with the benison of their wisdom, is always above reproach.

What if we were to look at *good faith* as *blind faith?*

Good faith, tenuous as skin-of-milk, is what sustains our nation. The slightest crack will plunge us into the abyss, and we dare not look close. But I think we should. We should trust our good sense and intelligence and face up to reality.

We are a fat nation, and we must examine *why* every time we purvey, prefer, prepare, present or partake in food.

Had I shared these horrors with those young chefs and mothers, their incredulity would have been swiftly replaced with redressal. They would have questioned me eagerly about the ingredients—what's safer, what's healthier.

What's tastier?

Nah, they hold the premium on that.

Their skills have made them supremely confident of making a new idea work. All they lack is information and opportunity.

Show us the impossible, and we cannot resist taking a shot at it.

Mired in the monumental stupidities of an invented past, we refuse to acknowledge the present, and totally disown the future. But hey, that's just political.

This is personal, deeply personal, and it doesn't get more politic than that.

Our decisions determine our health. They dictate our children's destiny.

In Corbett's time, the paratha would have been honest-to-goodness atta and desi ghee, and maybe, just maybe, you could face a man-eater on that. In today's jungle, that paratha is on the side of the man-eater, and unless we discern this in time, we are doomed not merely to suffer, but what's infinitely worse, to inflict suffering upon our children.

At the traffic light, I find myself between two buses, both emblazoned with advertisements.

To my left, a giant vada pao competes with the florid portrait of a politician.

To my right, a lingerie-clad beauty lounges in a slither of spaghetti and urges olive oil on me.

I fight free, resentfully.

Sadly, that is exactly where the public discourse on food is positioned—between gastro-politics and gastro-porn. And so it remains discredited, heaped with derision and scorn.

Isn't it time we rescued it?

Isn't it time we reclaimed the simple pleasures of intelligent eating, and demanded cheap, safe, delicious food as a basic Indian right?

That is all we need to stem the tide of obesity and diabetes.

That is all we need to do to keep the pale horseman from threatening our children dancing carefree in the rain.

References

The Body Blog

1. 'American Medical Association Adopts New Policies on Second Day of Voting at Annual Meeting' [Internet] 2013 [cited April 7, 2014]. Available from: http://www.ama-assn.org/ama/pub/news/news/2013/2013-06-18-new-ama-policies-annual-meeting.page.
2. Ng, Marie; Fleming, Tom; Robinson, Margaret; Thomson, Blake; Graetz, Nicholas; Margono, Christopher; Mullay, C.; Biryukov, Stan; Abbafati, Cristiana; Abera, Semae Ferede; Abraham, Jerry P.; Abu Rmeileh, Niveen M. E.; Achoki, Tom; Buhairan, Fadia S.A.I.; Alemu, Zewdie A.; Alfonso, Rafael; Kali, Mohammed; Ali, Raghib and Gakidou, Emmanuela.: 'Global, Regional, and National Prevalence of Overweight and Obesity in Children and Adults during 1980–2013: A systematic analysis for the Global Burden of Disease Study 2013' *The Lancet,* 30 August–5 September 2014; Volume 384, Issue 9945:766–78 doi: 10.1016/S0140-6736(14)60460–8
3. Sushruta. *Susruta Samhita—Sutrasthana,* Volume 1, Chapter XV:127
4. Hruby, Adela and Hu, Frank B.: 'The Epidemiology of Obesity: A big picture' *Pharmacoeconomics.* July 2015, 33(7):673–89.

Dermis Deluxe

1. Sun, Kai; Kusminski, Christine M. and Scherer, Philipp E.: 'Adipose Tissue Remodeling and Obesity' *Journal of Clinical Investigation,* 2011; 121(6):2094–101. doi: 10.1172/JCI45887.
2. Lee, Jane J; Pedley, Alison; Hoffmann, Udo; Massaro, Joseph M. and Fox, Caroline S.: 'Association of Changes in Abdominal Fat Quantity and Quality with Incident Cardiovascular Disease

Risk Factors' *Journal of the American College of Cardiology,* New York. October 4, 2016; 68.14:1509–21.

3. Arner, Peter; Bernard, Samuel; Salehpour, Mehran; Göran Possnert, Jakob Liebl; Steier, Peter; Buchholz, Bruce A.; Eriksson, Erik Arner Mats; Hauner, Hans; Skurk, Thomas; Mikael Rydén; Frayn, Keith N. and Spalding, Kirsty L.: 'Dynamics of Human Adipose Lipid Turnover in Health and Metabolic Disease' *Nature,* October 6, 2011; 478:110–13 doi: 10.1038/nature10426.
4. Lowe, Christopher E.; O'Rahilly, Stephen and Rochford, Justin J.: 'Adipogenesis at a Glance' *Journal of Cell Science,* 2011; 124:2681–6; doi: 10.1242/jcs.079699.
5. Iqbal, Jahangir and Hussain, M. Mahmood: 'Intestinal Lipid Absorption' *American Journal of Physiology–Endocrinology and Metabolism,* June 2009; 296(6):E1183–94. doi: 10.1152/ajpendo.90899.2008. Epub 2009 Jan 21.
6. Després, J.P.; Lemieux, I.; Bergeron, J.; Pibarot, P.; Mathieu, P.; Larose, E.; Rodés-Cabau, J.; Bertrand, O.F. and Poirier, P.: 'Abdominal Obesity and the Metabolic Syndrome: Contribution to global cardiometabolic risk' *Arteriosclerosis Thrombosis and Vascular Biology,* June 2008; 28(6):1039–49. doi: 10.1161/ATVBAHA.107.159228. Epub 2008 Mar 20.

The Changing Paradigm

1. The GBD 2015 Obesity Collaborators: 'Health Effects of Overweight and Obesity in 195 Countries over 25 Years' *New England Journal of Medicine,* July 6, 2017; 377:13–27 doi: 10.1056/NEJMoa1614362.
2. Jih, J.; Mukherjea, A.; Vittinghoff, E.; Nguyen, T.T.; Tsoh, J.Y.; Fukuoka, Y. and Kanaya, A.M.: 'Using Appropriate Body Mass Index Cut Points for Overweight and Obesity among Asian Americans' *Preventive Medicine*, 2014; 65:1–6. http://doi.org/10.1016/j.ypmed. 2014.04.010.
3. Palaniappan, L.P.; Araneta, M.R.G.; Assimes, T.L.; Barrett-Connor, E.L.; Carnethon, M.R.; Criqui, M.H. and Wong, N.D.: 'Call to Action: Cardiovascular Disease in Asian Americans: A science advisory from the American Heart Association' *Circulation,* 2010; 122(12):1242–52. doi: 10.1161/CIR.0b013e3181f22af4.

4. Mozaffarian, Dariush; Katan, Martijn B.; Ascherio, Alberto; Stampfer, Meir J. and Willett, Walter C.: 'Trans Fatty Acids and Cardiovascular Disease' *New England Journal of Medicine*, April 13, 2006; 354:1601–13 doi: 10.1056/ NEJMra054035
5. Lichtenstein, Alice H.: 'Trans Fatty Acids, Plasma Lipid Levels, and Risk of Developing Cardiovascular Disease. A statement for healthcare professionals from the American Heart Association' *Circulation*, 1997; 95:2588–90.

Measuring the Body

1. FAO, IFAD, UNICEF, WFP and WHO: *The State of Food Security and Nutrition in the World 2017. Building resilience for peace and food security*, 2017. Rome, FAO.
2. Mani, Indu and Kurpad, Anura V.: 'Fats & Fatty Acids in Indian Diets: Time for serious introspection' *The Indian Journal of Medical Research*, 2016; 144.4: 507–14. *PMC*. Web. 19 Oct. 2017.
3. Abarca-Gómez, Leandra et al.: 'Worldwide Trends in Body-Mass Index, Underweight, Overweight, and Obesity from 1975 to 2016: A pooled analysis of 2416 population-based measurement studies in 128·9 million children, adolescents, and adults' *The Lancet*, October 10, 2017; http://dx.doi.org/10.1016/ S0140-6736(17)32129-.
4. Hales, Craig M.; Carroll, Margaret D.; Fryar, Cheryl D. and Ogden, Cynthia L.: *Prevalence of Obesity Among Adults and Youth: United States, 2015–2016*, NCHS Data Brief No. 288, October 2017.
5. Björntorp, Per: 'Regional Patterns of Fat Distribution' *Annals of Internal Medicine*, 1985; 103:994–95. doi: 10.7326/0003-4819-103-6-994.
6. Larsson, B.; Svärdsudd, K.; Welin, L.; Wilhelmsen, L.; Björntorp, P.and Tibblin, G.: 'Abdominal Adipose Tissue Distribution, Obesity, and Risk of Cardiovascular Disease and Death: 13 year follow up of participants in the study of men born in 1913' *British Medical Journal* (Clinical Research Ed.), 1984; 288(6428):1401–4.
7. Balkau, B.; Deanfield, J.E.; Després, J.-P.; Bassan, J.-P.; Fox, K.A.A.; Smith, S.C. and Haffner, S.M.: 'International Day for the Evaluation of Abdominal Obesity (IDEA): A study

of waist circumference, cardiovascular disease, and diabetes mellitus in 168,000 primary care patients in 63 countries' *Circulation*, 2007; 116(17):1942–51. http://doi.org/ 10.1161/ CIRCULATIONAHA.106.676379.

8. Després, J.-P.; Arsenault, B.J.; Côté, M.; Cartier, A. and Lemieux, I.: 'Abdominal Obesity: The cholesterol of the 21st century?' *The Canadian Journal of Cardiology*, 2008; 24(Suppl D), 7D–12D.
9. Canoy, Dexter S; Boekholdt, Matthijs; Wareham, Nicholas; Luben, Robert; Welch, Ailsa; Bingham, Sheila; Buchan, Iain; Day, Nicholas and Khaw, Kay-Tee: 'Body Fat Distribution and Risk of Coronary Heart Disease in Men and Women in the European Prospective Investigation Into Cancer and Nutrition in Norfolk Cohort. A population-based prospective study' *Circulation*, December 18, 2007; 116(25):2933–43. Epub 2007 Dec 10.
10. Yusuf, Salim; Hawken, Steven; Ounpuu, Stephanie; Bautista, Leonelo; Franzosi, Maria Grazia; Commerford, Patrick; Lang, Chim; Rumboldt, Zvonko; Onen, Churchill L.; Lisheng, Liu; Tanomsup, Supachai; Wangai, Paul; Razak, Fahad; Sharma, Arya and Saad, Sonia: 'Obesity and the Risk of Myocardial Infarction in 27,000 Participants from 52 Countries: A case-control study' *The Lancet*, 2005; 366:1640–49. doi 10.1016/ S0140-6736(05)67663-5.
11. Pinho, Claudia Porto Sabino; Diniz, Alcides da Silva; de Arruda, Ilma Kruze Grande; Leite, Ana Paula Dornelas Leão; Petribú, Marina de Moraes Vasconcelos and Rodrigues, Isa Galvão: 'Predictive Models for Estimating Visceral Fat: The contribution from anthropometric parameters' *PLoS ONE*, 24 July, 2017; Vol. 12 Issue 7:1–12.
12. Brundavani, V.; Murthy, S R. and Kurpad, A.V.: 'Estimation of Deep Abdominal Adipose Tissue (DAAT) Accumulation from Simple Anthropometric Measurements in Indian Men and Women' *European Journal of Clinical Nutrition*, 2006; 60:658–66. doi 10.1038/sj.ejcn.1602366.
13. Shokeen, Deepa and Aeri, Bani Tamber: 'Prevalence of Cardio-Metabolic Risk Factors: A cross-sectional study among employed adults in urban Delhi, India' *Journal of Clinical and Diagnostic Research*, 2017; 11.8:LC01–LC04. *PMC*. Web. 19 Oct. 2017.

The Perfect Meal

1. Zusman, Oren; Theilla, Miriam; Cohen, Jonathan; Kagan, Ilya; Bendavid, Itai and Singer, Pierre: 'Resting Energy Expenditure, Calorie and Protein Consumption in Critically Ill Patients: A retrospective cohort study' *Critical Care*, 2016; 20:367. Published online Nov 10, 2016. doi: 10.1186/s13054-016-1538-4
2. Rao, Zhi-yong; Wu, Xiao-ting; Liang, Bin-miao; Wang, Mao-yun and Hu, Wen.: 'Comparison of Five Equations for Estimating Resting Energy Expenditure in Chinese Young, Normal Weight Healthy Adults' *European Journal of Medical Research*, 2012; 17(1):26. Published online September 1, 2012.

The Adipocyte at Home

1. Bartness, T.J.; Liu, Y.; Shrestha, Y.B. and Ryu, V.: 'Neural Innervation of White Adipose Tissue and the Control of Lipolysis' *Frontiers in Neuroendocrinology*, 2014; 35(4):473–93. doi: 10.1016/j.yfrne.2014.04.001.
2. Frayn, K.N.; Karpe, F.; Fielding, B.A.; Macdonald, I.A. and Coppack, S.W.: 'Integrative Physiology of Human Adipose Tissue' *International Journal of Obesity*, 2003; 27 (8):875–88.
3. Choe, S.S.; Huh, J.Y.; Hwang, I.J.; Kim, J.I. and Kim, J.B.: 'Adipose Tissue Remodeling: Its role in energy metabolism and metabolic disorders' *Frontiers in Endocrinology*, 2016; 7:30. doi: 10.3389/fendo.2016.00030.
4. Bjørndal, Bodil; Burri, Lena; Staalesen, Vidar; Skorve, Jon and Berge, Rolf K.: 'Different Adipose Depots: Their role in the development of metabolic syndrome and mitochondrial response to hypolipidemic agents' *Journal of Obesity*, 2011; vol. 2011, Article ID 490650, doi: 10.1155/2011/490650.
5. Bowles, L. and Kopelman, P.: 'Leptin: Of mice and men?' *Journal of Clinical Pathology*, 2001; 54(1):1–3. doi: 10.1136/jcp.54.1.1.
6. Zhang, Y.; Proenca, R.; Maffei, M.; Barone, M.; Leopold, L. and Friedman, J.M.: 'Positional Cloning of the Mouse Obese Gene and Its Human Homologue' *Nature*, 1994; 372:425–32.
7. Friedman, J.M.: 'A Conversation with Jeffrey M. Friedman by Ushma S. Neill' *Journal of Clinical Investigation*,

February 2013; 123(2):529–30.doi: 10.1172/JCI68394. Epub 2013 Feb 1.

8. Akoumianakis, Ioannis; Akawi, Nadia and Antoniades, Charalambos: 'Exploring the Crosstalk between Adipose Tissue and the Cardiovascular System' *Korean Circulation Journal,* September 2017; 47(5):670–85. doi: 10.4070/kcj.2017.0041. Epub 2017 Sep 21.
9. Giridharan, N.V.: 'Animal Models of Obesity & Their Usefulness in Molecular Approach to Obesity' *Indian Journal of Medical Research,* November 1998; 108:225–42.
10. Carroll, L.; Voisey, J. and van Daal, A.: 'Mouse Models of Obesity' *Clinical Dermatology*, July–August 2004; 22(4):345–9.
11. Ghosha, S; Swain, U.; Giridharan, N.V. and Raghunatha, M.: 'Increased Macromolecular Damage Due to Oxidative Stress in the Neocortex and Hippocampus of WNIN/Ob: A novel rat model of premature aging' *Neuroscience,* 6 June 2014; Volume 269:256–64

Metabolic Syndrome

1. Le, Ngoc Hoan; Kim , Chu-Sook; Tu, Thai Hien; Kim, Byung-Sam; Park, Taesun; Park, Jung Han Yoon; Goto, Tsuyoshi; Kawada, Teruo; Ha, Tae Youl and Yu, Rina: 'Absence of 4-1BB Reduces Obesity-Induced Atrophic Response in Skeletal Muscle' *Journal of Inflammation*, 2017; 14:9. Published online 2017 May 11. doi: 10.1186/s12950-017-0156-5.
2. Reddy, K.S.; Prabhakaran, D.; Chaturvedi, V.; Jeemon, P.; Thankappan, K.R.; Ramakrishnan, L.; Mohan, B.V.M.; Pandav, C.S.; Ahmed, F.U.: Joshi, P.P.; Meera, R.; Amin, R.B.; Ahuja, R.C.; Das, M.S. and Jaison, T.M.: 'Methods for Establishing a Surveillance System for Cardiovascular Diseases in Indian Industrial Populations' *Bulletin of the World Health Organization*, 2006; 84(6):461–69. https://dx.doi.org/10.1590/S0042-96862006000600015.
3. Reaven, Gerald M.: 'Role of Insulin Resistance in Human Disease' *Diabetes,* December 1988; 37(12):1595–1607; doi: 10.2337/diab.37.12.1595.
4. Meshram, Indrapal; Vardhana, Vishnu; Rao, M.; Vemula, Sudershan; Laxmaiah, Avula and Polasa, K.: 'Regional Variation

in the Prevalence of Overweight/Obesity, Hypertension and Diabetes and Their Correlates among the Adult Rural Population in India' *The British Journal of Nutrition*, 2016; -1:1–8. doi 10.1017/S0007114516000039.

5. DeMarco, V.G.; Aroor, A.R. and Sowers, J.R.: 'The Pathophysiology of Hypertension in Patients with Obesity' Nature Reviews in *Endocrinology*, 2014; 10(6):364–76. http://doi.org/ 10.1038/nrendo.2014.44.
6. Jo, J.; Gavrilova, O.; Pack, S. et al. 'Hypertrophy and/or Hyperplasia: Dynamics of adipose tissue growth' Papin, J.A., ed. *PLoS Computational Biology*, 2009; 5(3):e1000324. doi: 10.1371/journal.pcbi.1000324.
7. Gupta, R.; Guptha, S.; Agrawal, A.; Kaul, V.; Gaur, K. and Gupta, V.P.: 'Secular Trends in Cholesterol Lipoproteins and Triglycerides and Prevalence of Dyslipidemias in an Urban Indian Population' *Lipids in Health and Disease*, 2008; 7:40. doi: 10.1186/1476-511X-7-40.
8. Enas, E.A.; Garg, A.; Davidson, M.A.; Nair, V.M.; Huet, B.A. and Yusuf, S.: 'Coronary Heart Disease and Its Risk Factors in First-Generation Immigrant Asian Indians to the United States of America' *Indian Heart Journal*, July–August 1996; 48(4):343–53.
9. Gupta, Rajeev; Guptha, Soneil; Sharma, Krishna; Gupta, Arvind and Deedwania, Prakash.: 'Regional Variations in Cardiovascular Risk Factors in India: India Heart Watch' *World Journal of Cardiology*, 2012; 4:112–20. doi 10.4330/wjc.v4.i4.112.
10. Prasad, D.S.; Kabir, Z.; Dash, A.K. and Das, B.C.: 'Prevalence and Risk Factors for Metabolic Syndrome in Asian Indians: A community study from urban Eastern India' *Journal of Cardiovascular Disease Research*, 2012; 3(3):204–11. http://doi.org/ 10.4103/0975-3583.98895.

Bon Appetit!

1. Stokes, Jason W.; Boehm, Michael and Baier, Stefan.: 'Oral Processing, Texture and Mouthfeel: From rheology to tribology and beyond;' Current Opinion in *Colloid & Interface Science*. 2013; 18:349–59. 10.1016/j.cocis.2013.04.010.
2. Low, Yu Qing; Lacy, Kathleen and Keast, Russell: 'The Role

of Sweet Taste in Satiation and Satiety' *Nutrients,* 2014; 6.9: 3431–50. *PMC.* Web. 30 Oct. 2017.

3. Volkow, Nora D.; Wang, Gene-Jack and Baler, Ruben D.: 'Reward, Dopamine and the Control of Food Intake: Implications for obesity' *Trends in Cognitive Sciences,* 2011; 15.1:37–46. *PMC.* Web. 30 Oct. 2017.
4. Cassidy, Ryan Michael and Tong, Qingchun: 'Hunger and Satiety Gauge Reward Sensitivity' *Frontiers in Endocrinology,* 2017; 8:104. *PMC.* Web. 30 Oct. 2017
5. Druce, M. and Bloom, S.R.: 'The Regulation of Appetite' *Archives of Disease in Childhood,* 2006; 91(2):183–7. doi: 10.1136/adc.2005.073759.

The Taste of Fat

1. Sherwin, R.: 'Controlled Trials of the Diet-Heart Hypothesis: Some comments on the experimental unit' *America Journal of Epidemiology,* 1978; 108:92–9.
2. Executive Committee on Diet and Heart Disease. *National Diet-Heart Study Report.* American Heart Association, 1968.
3. Ramsden, C.E.; Zamora, D; Leelarthaepin, B.; Majchrzak-Hong, S.F.; Faurot, K.R.; Suchindran, C.M.; Ringel, A.; Davis, J.M. and Hibbeln, J.R.: 'Use of Dietary Linoleic Acid for Secondary Prevention of Coronary Heart Disease and Death: Evaluation of recovered data from the Sydney Diet Heart Study and updated meta-analysis' *British Medical Journal,* February 4, 2013; 346:e8707. doi: 10.1136/bmj.e8707.
4. Ramsden, Christopher E.; Zamora, Daisy; Majchrzak-Hong, Sharon; Faurot, Keturah R.; Broste, Steven K;. Frantz, Robert P.; Davis, John M.; Ringel, Amit; Suchindran, Chirayath M. and Hibbeln, Joseph R.: 'Re-evaluation of the Traditional Diet-Heart Hypothesis: Analysis of recovered data from Minnesota Coronary Experiment (1968-73)' *British Medical Journal,* April 12, 2016; 353 doi: https://doi.org/10.1136/bmj.i1246
5. Directorate of Vanaspati, Vegetable Oil and Fats (DVVOF): *Commodity Profile of Edible Oil for December—2016;* agricoop.gov.in/sites/default/files/edib_2201.pdf.
6. Mani, Indu, and Kurpad, Anura V.: 'Fats & Fatty Acids in Indian Diets: Time for serious introspection' *The Indian Journal of Medical Research,* 2016; 144.4:507–14. *PMC.* Web. 31 Oct. 2017.

7. Indian Council of Medical Research. *Nutrient Requirements and Recommended Dietary Allowances for Indians*. Report of the Expert Group of the Indian Council of Medical Research. Hyderabad: National Institute of Nutrition; 2010.
8. Deol, P; Evans, J.R.; Dhahbi, J.; Chellappa, K.; Han, D.S.; Spindler, S. et al.: 'Soybean Oil Is More Obesogenic and Diabetogenic than Coconut Oil and Fructose in Mouse: Potential role for the liver.' *PLoS ONE*, 2015; 10(7):e0132672. https://doi.org/10.1371/journal.pone. 0132672.
9. Pimpin, Laura; Wu, Jason H. Y.; Haskelberg, Hila; Del Gobbo, Liana and Mozaffarian, Dariush: 'Is Butter Back? A systematic review and meta-analysis of butter consumption and risk of cardiovascular disease, diabetes, and total mortality' *PLoS ONE*, June 29, 2016; https://doi.org/10.1371/journal.pone.0158118.
10. Willett, W.C.: 'Trans Fatty Acids and Cardiovascular Disease—Epidemiological data' *Atherosclerosis Supplements,* May 2006, Volume 7, Issue 2:5–8.
11. Mozaffarian, D.; Katan, M.B.; Ascherio, A.; Stampfer, M.J. and Willett, W.C.: 'Trans Fatty Acids and Cardiovascular Disease' *New England Journal of Medicine,* 13 April 2006; 354(15):1601–13.
12. Ghosh-Jerath, Suparna: *Transfats in Indian Food Supply, From Production to Consumption—A case study from North India.* Indian Institute of Public Health, Delhi Public Health Foundation. http://www.iiasa.sc.at/Admin/PUB/Documents/WP-95-061.
13. Simopoulos, A.P.: 'An Increase in the Omega-6/Omega-3 Fatty Acid Ratio Increases the Risk for Obesity' *Nutrients,* 2016; 8(3):128. doi: 10.3390/nu8030128.

This, That, and the Other

1. MacDougall, Duncan: 'Hypothesis Concerning Soul Substance Together With Experimental Evidence of the Existence of Such a Substance' *Journal of the American Society for Psychical Research*, 1907; 1(1):237.
2. MacDougall, Duncan: 'The Soul: Hypothesis: Concerning soul substance together with experimental evidence of the existence of such substance' *American Medicine,* April 1907; 2:240–43.

3. Deeming, D. Charles and Pike, Thomas W.: 'Embryonic Growth and Antioxidant Provision in Avian Eggs' *Biology Letters,* 9.6 (2013): 20130757. *PMC*. Web. 6 Nov. 2017.
4. Yilmaz, B.; Sahin, K.; Bilen, H.; Bahcecioglu, I.H.; Bilir, B.; Ashraf, S. and Kucuk, O.: 'Carotenoids and Non-Alcoholic Fatty Liver Disease' *Hepatobiliary Surgery and Nutrition*, 2015; 4(3):161–71. http://doi.org/10.3978/j.issn.2304-3881.2015.01.11.
5. Fabbrini, Elisa; Sullivan, Shelby and Klein, Samuel: 'Obesity and Non-Alcoholic Fatty Liver Disease: Biochemical, metabolic and clinical implications' *Hepatology*, 2010; 51.2:679–89. *PMC*. Web. 6 Nov. 2017.
6. Das, Bhabatosh; Ghosh, Tarini Shankar; Kedia, Saurabh; Rampal, Ritika; Saxena, Shruti; Bag, Satyabrata; Mitra, Ridhima; Dayal, Mayanka; Mehta, Ojasvi; Surendranath, A.; Travis, Simon P.L.; Tripathi, Prabhanshu; Nair, G. Balakrish and Ahuja, Vineet. 'Analysis of the Gut Microbiome of Rural and Urban Healthy Indians Living in Sea Level and High Altitude Areas' *Nature Scientific Reports,* July 4, 2018; volume 8, article number 10104
7. Bhute, S.; Pande, P.; Shetty, S.A.; Shelar, R.; Mane, S.; Kumbhare, S.V.; Gawali, A.; Makhani, H.; Navandar, M.; Dhotre, D.; Lubree, H.; Agarwal, D.; Patil, R.; Ozarkar, S.; Ghaskadbi, S.; Yajnik, C.; Juvekar, S.; Makharia, G.K. and Shouche, Y.S.: 'Molecular Characterization and Meta-Analysis of Gut Microbial Communities Illustrate Enrichment of Prevotella and Megasphaera in Indian Subjects' *Frontiers in Microbiology*, 2016; 7:660. doi: 10.3389/fmicb.2016.00660
8. Östh, M.; Öst, A,; Kjolhede, P. and Strålfors, P.: 'The Concentration of β-Carotene in Human Adipocytes, but Not the Whole-Body Adipocyte Stores, Is Reduced in Obesity' *PLoS ONE,* 2014; 9(1):e85610. https://doi.org/10.1371/journal.pone.0085610.
9. Jeyakumar, Shanmugam M. and Ayyalasomayajula, Vajreswari: 'Vitamin A as a Key Regulator of Obesity and its Associated Disorders: Evidences from an obese rat model' *Indian Journal of Medical Research,* March 2015; 141(3):275–84.
10. Sadasivaiah, S.; Tozan, Y. and Breman, J.G.: 'Dichlorodiphenyltrichloroethane (DDT) for Indoor Residual Spraying in Africa: How can it be used for malaria control?' in:

Breman, J.G.; Alilio, M.S. and White, N.J., editors, *Defining and Defeating the Intolerable Burden of Malaria III: Progress and perspectives: Supplement to volume 77(6) of American Journal of Tropical Medicine and Hygiene.* December 2007; Northbrook (IL): American Society of Tropical Medicine and Hygiene. Available from: https://www.ncbi.nlm.nih.gov/books/NBK1724/

11. Maurya, Ashok Kumar; Kumar, Anoop and Joseph, P.E.: 'Trends in Ambient Loads of DDT and HCH Residues in Animal's and Mother's Milk of Paliakalan Kheeri, Uttar Pradesh-India' *International Journal of Scientific and Research Publications*, May 2013; Volume 3, Issue 5:2250–3153
12. Basu, Soma: 'India Opposes 2020 Deadline for DDT Ban' in *Down to Earth*, July 4, 2015; https://www.downtoearth.org.in/news/india-opposes-2020-deadline-for-ddt-ban-40967
13. van den Berg, Henk: 'Global Status of DDT and Its Alternatives for Use in Vector Control to Prevent Disease' *Environmental Health Perspectives,* November 2009; 117(11):1656–63. Published online 2009 May 29. doi: 10.1289/ehp.0900785 PMCID: PMC2801202
14. Cohn, Barbara A.; La Merrill, Michele; Krigbaum, Nickilou Y.; Yeh, Gregory; Park, June-Soo; Zimmermann, Lauren and Cirillo, Piera M.: 'DDT Exposure in Utero and Breast Cancer' *Journal of Clinical Endocrinology Metabolism,* August 2015; 100(8):2865–72. doi: 10.1210/jc.2015-1841. Epub 2015 Jun 16.
15. Chevrier, J.; Dewailly, Eric; Ayotte, Pierre; Mauriège, Pascale; Després, Jean-Pierre and Tremblay, A.: 'Body Weight Loss Increases Plasma and Adipose Tissue Concentrations of Potentially Toxic Pollutants in Obese Individuals' *International Journal of Obesity and Related Metabolic Disorders: Journal of the International Association for the Study of Obesity*, 2010; 24:1272–8. 10.1038/sj.ijo.0801380.
16. Reaves, D.K.; Ginsburg, E.; Bang, J.J. and Fleming, J.M.: 'Persistent Organic Pollutants & Obesity: Potential mechanisms for breast cancer promotion?' *Endocrine-Related Cancer,* (2015); 22(2):R69–R86. http://doi.org/10.1530/ERC-14-0411.
17. Herrera, B.M.; Keildson, S. and Lindgren, C.M.: 'Genetics and Epigenetics of Obesity' *Maturitas,* 2011; 69(1):41–9. http://doi.org/10.1016/j.maturitas.2011.02.018.

18. Yajnik, C.S.; Fall, C.H.D.; Coyaji, K.J.; Hirve, S.S.; Rao, S.; Barker, D.J.P. et al.: 'Neonatal Anthropometry: The thin-fat Indian baby—The Pune maternal nutrition study' *International Journal of Obesity Related Metabolic Disord*ers, 2003; 27:173–80. doi: 10.1038/sj.ijo.802219

Sugar, Sugar, Everywhere

1. Stanhope, Kimber L.: 'Sugar Consumption, Metabolic Disease and Obesity: The state of the controversy' *Critical Reviews in Clinical Laboratory Sciences,* 2016; Vol. 53, Iss. 1:52–67 Published online: 17 Sep 2015.
2. Harington, Kate; Smeele, Rebecca; Van Loon, Fiona; Yuan, Jannee; Haszard, Jillian Joy; Drewer, Amanda and Venn, Bernard Joseph: 'Desire for Sweet Taste Unchanged After Eating: Evidence of a dessert mentality?' *Journal of the American College of Nutrition* 2016; 35:6:581–6.
3. Commodity Profile for Sugar, July 2017: http://agricoop.gov.in/sites/default/files/Sugar per cent20Profile per cent20July per cent202017.pdf.

The Quotidian

1. Siwicki, K.K.; Eastman, C.; Petersen, G.; Rosbash, M. and Hall, J.C.: 'Antibodies to the Period Gene Product of *Drosophila* Reveal Diverse Tissue Distribution and Rhythmic Changes in the Visual System' *Neuron,* 1998; 1:141–50.
2. Hardin, P.E.; Hall, J.C. and Rosbash, M.: 'Feedback of the *Drosophila* Period Gene Product on Circadian Cycling of its Messenger RNA levels' *Nature,* 1990; 343:536–40.
3. The Nobel Assembly at Karolinska Institutet: Announcement of the 2017 Nobel Prize in Physiology or Medicine. https://assets.nobelprize.org/uploads/2018/06/press-39.pdf?_ga=2.173384419.1988868705.1537350900-983137122.1537350900

Breakfast on the Street

1. Maillard, L.C.: 'Action of Amino Acids on Sugars: Formation of melanoidins in a methodical way' *Comptes Rendus Chimie,* 1912; 154:66–8.

Rice Stories

1. Mayberry, Jessica: 'One Death, Three Stories About Sickness and Starvation in Jharkhand' thewire.in, 16 November 2017; https://thewire.in/197238/jharkhand-starvation-death-media-politics/
2. Johari, Aarefa: 'Denied food because she did not have Aadhaar-linked ration card, Jharkhand girl dies of starvation' Scroll.in, Oct 16, 2017; https://scroll.in/article/854225/denied-food-because-she-did-not-have-aadhaar-linked-ration-card-jharkhand-girl-dies-of-starvation.

The Body Politic: The Brain's Story

1. Hitze, B.; Hubold, C.; van Dyken, R.; Schlichting, K.; Lehnert, H.; Entringer, S. and Peters, A.: 'How the Selfish Brain Organizes its Supply and Demand' *Frontiers in Neuroenergetics*, 2010; 2, 7. http://doi.org/10.3389/fnene.2010.00007.
2. Peters, A. and Langemann, D.: 'Build-Ups in the Supply Chain of the Brain: On the neuroenergetic cause of obesity and type 2 diabetes mellitus' *Frontiers in Neuroenergetics*, 2009; 1, 2. http://doi.org/10.3389/neuro.14.002.2009.
3. Suzuki, Keisuke; Jayasena, Channa N. and Bloom, Stephen R.: 'The Gut Hormones in Appetite Regulation' *Journal of Obesity*, vol. 2011, Article ID 528401, https://doi.org/ 10.1155/2011/528401
4. Berthoud, H.-R. and Münzberg, H. 'The Lateral Hypothalamus as Integrator of Metabolic and Environmental Needs: From electrical self-stimulation to opto-genetics' *Physiology & Behaviour*, 2011; 104(1):29–39. doi: 10.1016/j.physbeh.2011.04.051.
5. Louis, G.W.; Leinninger, GRAMMES; Rhodes, C.J.; Myers, M.G.; 'Direct Innervation and Modulation of Orexin Neurons by Lateral Hypothalamic Leprb Neurons' *The Journal of Neuroscience: The official journal of the Society for Neuroscience*, 2010; 30(34):11278–87. doi: 10.1523/JNEUROSCI.1340-10.2010.
6. Morton, G.J.; Meek, T.H. and Schwartz, M.W.: 'Neurobiology of Food Intake in Health and Disease' Nature Reviews in *Neuroscience,* 2014; 15(6):367–78. doi: 10.1038/nrn3745.

7. Barateiro, A.; Mahú, I. and Domingos, A.I.: 'Leptin Resistance and the Neuro-Adipose Connection' *Frontiers in Endocrinology,* 2017; 8:45. doi: 10.3389/fendo.2017.00045.
8. Thon, M., Hosoi, T. and Ozawa, K.: 'Possible Integrative Actions of Leptin and Insulin Signaling in the Hypothalamus Targeting Energy Homeostasis' *Frontiers in Endocrinology,* 2016; 7:138. doi: 10.3389/fendo.2016.00138.

The Body Politic: The Cormorant Stomach

1. Chen, Jing; Chen, Lihong; Sanseau, Philippe; Freudenberg, Johannes M. and Rajpal, Deepak K.: 'Significant Obesity Associated Gene Expression Changes Occur in the Stomach but not Intestines in Obese Mice' *Physiological Reports,* May 2016; 4(10):e12793. Published online 2016 May 20. doi: 10.14814/phy2.12793
2. Saqui-Salces, Milena; Dowdle, William E.; Reiter, Jeremy F. and Merchant, Juanita L.: 'A High-Fat Diet Regulates Gastrin and Acid Secretion through Primary Cilia' *The FASEB Journal,* August 2012; 26(8):3127–39. doi: 10.1096/fj.11-197426

The Body Politic: The Liver

1. de Lartigue, G.: 'Role of the Vagus Nerve in the Development and Treatment of Diet-Induced Obesity' *Journal of Physiology,* 2016; 594:5791–815. doi: 10.1113/JP27153.
2. Catanzaro, R.; Cuffari, B.; Italia, A. and Marotta, F.: 'Exploring the Metabolic Syndrome: Non-alcoholic fatty pancreas disease' *World Journal of Gastroenterology,* 2016; 22(34):7660–75. http://doi.org/10.3748/wjg.v22.i34.7660.
3. Arslan, Nur: 'Obesity, Fatty Liver Disease and Intestinal Microbiota' *World Journal of Gastroenterology,* 2014; 20.44: 16452–63. *PMC.* Web. 30 Nov. 2017.
4. Gill, Harjot K. and Wu, George Y.: 'Non-Alcoholic Fatty Liver Disease and the Metabolic Syndrome: Effects of weight loss and a review of popular diets. Are low carbohydrate diets the answer?' *World Journal of Gastroenterology,* January 21, 2006; 12(3):345–53. PMCID: PMC4066051 Published online 2006 Jan 21. doi: 10.3748/wjg.v12.i3.345.
5. Kitade, Hironori; Chen, Guanliang; Ni, Yinhua and Ota, Tsuguhito: 'Non-alcoholic Fatty Liver Disease and Insulin

Resistance: New insights and potential new treatments' *Nutrients,* April 2017; 9(4):387. PMCID: PMC5409726 Published online 2017 Apr 14. doi: 10.3390/nu9040387.

6. Patell, R.; Dosi, R.; Joshi, H.; Sheth, S.; Shah, P. and Jasdanwala, S.: 'Non-Alcoholic Fatty Liver Disease (NAFLD) in Obesity' *Journal of Clinical and Diagnostic Research*, 2014; 8(1):62–6. doi: 10.7860/JCDR/2014/6691.3953.
7. Ajmal, M.R.; Yaccha, M.; Malik, M.A.; Rabbani, M.U.; Ahmad, I.; Isalm, N. and Abdali, N.: 'Prevalence of Non-Alcoholic Fatty Liver Disease (NAFLD) in Patients of Cardiovascular Diseases and Its Association with hs-CRP and TNF- ' *Indian Heart Journal*, 2014; 66(6):574–9. http://doi.org/10.1016/j.ihj.2014.08.006.
8. Wong, Robert J. and Ahmed, Aijaz: 'Obesity and Non-Alcoholic Fatty Liver Disease: Disparate Associations among Asian Populations' *World Journal of Hepatology*, 2014; 6.5: 263–73. *PMC*. Web. 30 Nov. 2017.
9. Erlinger, S.: 'Gallstones in Obesity and Weight Loss' *European Journal of Gastroenterology and Hepatology*, December 2000; 12(12):1347–52.
10. Liu, J.; Han, L.; Zhu, L. and Yu, Y.: 'Free Fatty Acids, Not Triglycerides, Are Associated with Non-Alcoholic Liver Injury Progression in High Fat Diet Induced Obese Rats' *Lipids in Health and Disease*, 2016; 15:27. doi: 10.1186/s12944-016-0194-7.

The Body Politic: Our Steed the Leg

1. Egan, Brendan; Zierath, Juleen R.: 'Exercise Metabolism and the Molecular Regulation of Skeletal Muscle Adaptation' *Cell Metabolism,* February 5, 2013; 17(2):162–84
2. Summermatter, Serge and Handschin, C.: 'PGC-1α and Exercise in the Control of Body Weight' *International Journal of Obesity* (2005). 2012; 36. doi 10.1038/ijo.2012.12.
3. Golbidi, Saeid; Mesdaghinia, A. and Laher, Ismail: 'Exercise in the Metabolic Syndrome' *Oxidative Medicine and Cellular Longevity,* 2012. 349710. doi 10.1155/2012/349710.
4. Mudry, J.M.; Massart, J.; Szekeres, F.L. and Krook, A.: 'TWIST1 and TWIST2 Regulate Glycogen Storage and Inflammatory Genes in Skeletal Muscle' *Journal of Endocrinology,* March 2015; 224(3):303–13. doi: 10.1530/JOE-14-0474.

5. Mudry, J.M.; Alm, P.S.; Erhardt, S.; Goiny, M.; Fritz, T.; Caidahl, K.; Zierath, J.R.; Krook, A. and Wallberg-Henriksson, H.: 'Direct Effects of Exercise on Kynurenine Metabolism in People with Normal Glucose Tolerance or Type 2 Diabetes' *Diabetes Metabolism Research and Reviews,* March 4, 2016; doi: 10.1002/dmrr.2798.
6. Mudry, J.M.; Kirchner, H.; Chibalin, A.V.; Krook, A. and Zierath, J.R.: 'Changes in Skeletal Muscle DNA Methylation in Rats Following Endurance Training and High-Fat Diet'. In manuscript.
7. Mudry, J.M.; Lassiter, D.G.; Nylén, C.; García-Calzón, S.; Näslund, E.; Krook, A. and Zierath, J.R.: 'Insulin and Glucose Alter Death-Associated Protein Kinase 3 (DAPK3) DNA Methylation in Human Skeletal Muscle' Manuscript under revision.
8. Tomlinson, D.J.; Erskine, R.M.; Winwood, K.; Morse, C.I. and Onambélé, G.L.: 'The Impact of Obesity on Skeletal Muscle Architecture in Untrained Young vs. Old Women' *Journal of Anatomy*, 2014; 225:675–84. doi: 10.1111/joa.12248
9. Neel, J.V : 'Diabetes Mellitus: A "thrifty" genotype rendered detrimental by "progress"?' *American Journal of Human Genetics,* 1996; 14(4):353–62. *PMC* 1932342. PMID 1393788
10. Neel, J.V.: 'The "Thrifty Genotype" in 1998' *Nutrition Reviews,* 2009; 57(5):2–9. doi: 10.1111/j.1753-4887.1999.tb01782.x. PMID 10391020.

The Body Politic: Shadow Play—The Micobiome

1. Toribio-Mateas, Miguel. 'Harnessing the Power of Microbiome Assessment Tools as Part of Neuroprotective Nutrition and Lifestyle Medicine Interventions' *Microorganisms,* 2018; 6.2:35.
2. Nehra, V.; Allen, J.M.; Mailing, L.J.; Kashyap, P.C. and Woods, J.A.: 'Gut Microbiota: Modulation of host physiology in obesity' *Physiology*, 2016; 31(5):327–35. doi: 10.1152/physiol.00005.2016.

The Body Politic: High Blood Pressure

1. Babu, G.R.; Murthy, G.V.S.; Ana, Y.; Patel, P.; Deepa, R.; Neelon, S.E.B. and Reddy, K.S.: 'Association of Obesity with

Hypertension and Type 2 Diabetes Mellitus in India: A meta-analysis of observational studies' *World Journal of Diabetes*, 2018; 9(1):40–52. http://doi.org/10.4239/wjd.v9.i1.40.
2. Tripathy, J.P.; Thakur, J.S.; Jeet, G.; Chawla, S. and Jain, S.: 'Alarmingly High Prevalence of Hypertension and Pre-Hypertension in North India: Results from a large cross-sectional STEPS survey' *PLoS ONE*, 2017; 12(12):e0188619. https://doi.org/10.1371/journal.pone.0188619.
3. DeMarco, V.G.; Aroor, A.R. and Sowers, J.R.: 'The Pathophysiology of Hypertension in Patients with Obesity' Nature Reviews in *Endocrinology*, 2014; 10(6):364–76. doi: 10.1038/nrendo.2014.44.

A 'Civilization Syndrome'

1. Van der Valk, E.S.; Savas, M. and van Rossum, E.F.C.: 'Stress and Obesity: Are there more susceptible individuals?' *Current Obesity Reports*, 2018; 7(2):193–203. http://doi.org/10.1007/s13679-018-0306-y.
2. Kyrou, Ioannis; Chrousos, George P. and Tsigos, Constantine: 'Stress, Visceral Obesity, and Metabolic Complications' *Annals of the New York Academy of Sciences,* November 17, 2006; Volume 1083, Issue 1; https://doi.org/10.1196/annals.1367.008.
3. Bose, Mousumi; Oliván, Blanca and Laferrère, Blandine: 'Stress and Obesity: The role of the hypothalamic–pituitary–adrenal axis in metabolic disease' *Current Opinion in Endocrinology, Diabetes, and Obesity*, 2009; 16.5:340–46.
4. Hirotsu, Camila; Tufik, Sergio and Andersen, Monica Levy: 'Interactions between Sleep, Stress, and Metabolism: From physiological to pathological conditions' *Sleep Science*, 2015; 8.3:143–52.
5. Björntorp, Per: 'Visceral Obesity: A "civilization syndrome"' *Obesity Research and Clinical Practice,* May 1993; 1(3):206–22.
6. Krishnaveni, G.V.; Jones, A.; Veena, S.R.; Somashekara, R.; Karat, S.C.D. and Fall, C.H.: 'Adiposity and Cortisol Response to Stress in Indian Adolescents' *Indian Paediatrics,* February 15, 2018; 55(2):125–30. Epub 2017 Dec 14.
7. Peeke, P.M. and Chrousos, G.P.: 'Hypercortisolism and Obesity' *Annals of the New York Academy of Sciences,* 1995; 771:665–76.

8. Goldstein, David S.: 'Adrenal Responses to Stress' *Cellular and Molecular Neurobiology*, 2010; 30.8:1433–40.
9. Cannon, W.B.: 'Organization for Physiological Homeostasis' *Physiological Reviews*, 1929a; 9:399–431.
10. Cannon, Walter B.: *Bodily Changes in Pain, Hunger, Fear and Rage,* New York: D. Appleton & Co., 1929.
11. Selye, Hans: *Stress without Distress,* New American Library; New York: 1974.

The State of the Nation

1. Indian Council of Medical Research, Public Health Foundation of India, and Institute for Health Metrics and Evaluation. *India: Health of the Nation's States—The India State-level Disease Burden Initiative*. New Delhi, India: ICMR, PHFI, and IHME; 2017.
2. 'Nations Within a Nation: Variations in epidemiological transition across the states of India, 1990–2016 in the Global Burden of Disease Study'; India State-level Disease Burden Initiative Collaborators; *The Lancet*, Volume 390, Issue 10111:2437–460. [Lalit Dandona, Rakhi Dandona, G. Anil Kumar, D.K. Shukla, Vinod K. Paul, Kalpana Balakrishnan, Dorairaj Prabhakaran, Nikhil Tandon, Sundeep Salvi, A.P. Dash, A. Nandakumar, Vikram Patel, Sanjay K. Agarwal, Prakash C. Gupta, R.S. Dhaliwal, Prashant Mathur, Avula Laxmaiah, Preet K. Dhillon, Subhojit Dey, Manu R. Mathur, Ashkan Afshin, Christina Fitzmaurice, Emmanuela Gakidou, Peter Gething, Simon I. Hay, Nicholas J. Kassebaum, Hmwe Kyu, Stephen S. Lim, Mohsen Naghavi, Gregory A. Roth, Jeffrey D. Stanaway, Harvey Whiteford, Vineet K. Chadha, Sunil D. Khaparde, Raghuram Rao, Kirankumar Rade, Puneet Dewan, Melissa Furtado, Eliza Dutta, Chris M. Varghese, Ravi Mehrotra, P. Jambulingam, Tanvir Kaur, Meenakshi Sharma, Shalini Singh, Rashmi Arora, Reeta Rasaily, Ranjit M. Anjana, Viswanathan Mohan, Anurag Agrawal, Arvind Chopra, Ashish J. Mathew, Deeksha Bhardwaj, Pallavi Muraleedharan, Parul Mutreja, Kelly Bienhoff, Scott Glenn, Rizwan S. Abdulkader, Ashutosh N. Aggarwal, Rakesh Aggarwal, Sandra Albert, Atul Ambekar, Monika Arora, Damodar Bachani, Ashish Bavdekar, Gufran Beig, Anil Bhansali, Anurag Bhargava, Eesh Bhatia,

Bilali Camara, D.J. Christopher, Siddharth K. Das, Paresh V. Dave, Sagnik Dey, Aloke G. Ghoshal, N. Gopalakrishnan, Randeep Guleria, Rajeev Gupta, Subodh S. Gupta, Tarun Gupta, M.D. Gupte, G. Gururaj, Sivadasanpillai Harikrishnan, Veena Iyer, Sudhir K. Jain, Panniyamamkal Jeemon, Vasna Joshua, Rajni Kant, Anita Kar, Amal C. Kataki, Kiran Katoch, Ajay Khera, Sanjay Kinra, Parvaiz A. Koul, Anand Krishnan, Avdhesh Kumar, Raman K. Kumar, Rashmi Kumar, Anura Kurpad, Laishram Ladusingh, Rakesh Lodha, P.A. Mahesh, Rajesh Malhotra, Matthews Mathai, Dileep Mavalankar, Murali Mohan B.V., Satinath Mukhopadhyay, Manoj Murhekar, G.V.S. Murthy, Sanjeev Nair, Sreenivas A. Nair, Lipika Nanda, Romi S. Nongmaithem, Anu M. Oommen, Jeyaraj D. Pandian, Sapan Pandya, Sreejith Parameswaran, Sanghamitra Pati, Kameshwar Prasad, Narayan Prasad, Manorama Purwar, Asma Rahim, Sreebhushan Raju, Siddarth Ramji, Thara Rangaswamy, Goura K. Rath, Ambuj Roy, Yogesh Sabde, K.S. Sachdeva, Harsiddha Sadhu, Rajesh Sagar, Mari J. Sankar, Rajendra Sharma, Anita Shet, Shreya Shirude, Rajan Shukla, Sharvari R. Shukla, Gagandeep Singh, Narinder P. Singh, Virendra Singh, Anju Sinha, Dhirendra N. Sinha, R.K. Srivastava, A. Srividya, Vanita Suri, Rajaraman Swaminathan, P.N. Sylaja, Babasaheb Tandale, J.S. Thakur, Kavumpurathu R. Thankappan, Nihal Thomas, Srikanth Tripathy, Mathew Varghese, Santosh Varughese, S. Venkatesh, K. Venugopal, Lakshmi Vijayakumar, Denis Xavier, Chittaranjan S. Yajnik, Geevar Zachariah, Sanjay Zodpey, J.V.R. Prasada Rao, Theo Vos, K. Srinath Reddy, Christopher J.L. Murray, Soumya Swaminathan]

3. 'The Increasing Burden of Diabetes and Variations Among the States of India: The Global Burden of Disease Study 1990–2016' *India State-Level Disease Burden Initiative Diabetes Collaborators* www.thelancet.com/lancetgh Published online September 12, 2018 http://dx.doi.org/10.1016/S2214-109X(18)30387-5 1

Ours to Reason Why

1. http://www.diabetesatlas.org/across-the-globe.html
2. http://www.diabetesatlas.org

3. http://agricoop.gov.in/sites/default/files/Edible%20oil%20 Profile%2026-04-2018.pdf
4. Giacconea, Vita; Cammilleria, Gaetano; Di Stefanob, Vita; Pitonzoc, Rosa; Vellaa, Antonio; Pulvirentid, Andrea; Lo Dicoa, Gianluigi Maria; Ferrantellia, Vincenzo and Macaluso, Andrea: 'First Report on the Presence of Alloxan in Bleached Flour by LC-MS/MS Method' *Journal of Cereal Science,* September 2017; Volume 77:120–25
5. https://toxnet.nlm.nih.gov/cgi-bin/sis/search/a?dbs+hsdb:@ term+@DOCNO+7493
6. McLuhan, Marshall. 'McLuhan: Now The Medium Is The Massage' *New York Times,* 1967-03-19
7. Alfred, Lord Tennyson. 'The Charge of the Light Brigade' 1854.

Solutions

1. März, W.; Kleber, M.E.; Scharnagl, H. et al.: 'HDL Cholesterol: Reappraisal of its clinical relevance' *Clinical Research in Cardiology*, 2017; 106(9):663–75. doi: 10.1007/s00392-017-1106-1.
2. Traversy, G. and Chaput, J.-P.: 'Alcohol Consumption and Obesity: An update' *Current Obesity Reports*, 2015; 4(1):122–30. doi: 10.1007/s13679-014-0129-4.

The Pale Horseman

1. Solomon, Harris: *Metabolic Living—Food, fat, and the absorption of illness in India*; Duke University Press; 2016.
2. Purba, M.K.; Agrawal, N. and Shukla, S.K.: 'Detection of Non-Permitted Food Colours in Edibles' *Journal of Forensic Research,* 2015; S4:003. doi: 10.4172/2157-7145.1000S4-003.
3. Accum, Fredrick: *A Treatise on Adulterations of Food, and Culinary Poisons—Exhibiting the fraudulent sophistications of bread, beer, wine, spirituous liquors, tea, oil, pickles, and other articles employed in domestic economy. And methods of detecting them;* Longman, Hurst, Rees, Orme, and Brown, London; 1820.

Index